Healthcare Interpreting in Small Bites

50 Nourishing Selections from the "Pacific Interpreters Newsletter," 2002-2010

by Cynthia E. Roat

Published by

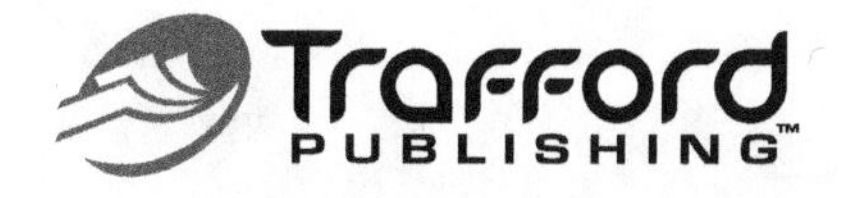

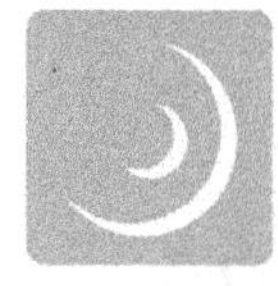

Disclaimer

This product is intended to offer advice and guidance on the skills and techniques of interpreting in the healthcare environment. It is not intended to teach medicine, give medical advice, or promote any skill other than interpreting and translating. While every effort has been made to use terminology, descriptions and examples that are realistic and accurate, we make absolutely no representations as to the medical content of this book. Medical advice, medical opinions, and apparent statements of medical fact are intended only to provide readers with plausible context for discussion of interpretation and translation. In no case should they construed as actual advice, opinion, or statements of medical professionals; they are not. Do not use this book as a guide to medical action.

All puzzles constructed at www.puzzlemaker.com.
Cover design and interior layout by Grinning Moon Creative, www.grinningmoon.com.

Healthcare Interpreting in Small Bites

50 Nourishing Selections from the "Pacific Interpreters Newsletter," 2002-2010

by Cynthia E. Roat

Order this book online at www.trafford.com
or email orders@trafford.com

Most Trafford titles are also available at major online book retailers.

Printed in the United States of America.

ISBN: 978-1-4269-3122-2 (sc)

Library of Congress Control Number: 2010905173

Our mission is to efficiently provide the world's finest, most comprehensive book publishing service, enabling every author to experience success. To find out how to publish your book, your way, and have it available worldwide, visit us online at www.trafford.com

Trafford rev. 11/08/2010

Trafford PUBLISHING www.trafford.com

North America & international
toll-free: 1 888 232 4444 (USA & Canada)
phone: 250 383 6864 • fax: 812 355 4082

Acknowledgements

We are especially grateful to the following individuals who assisted with this project: for their advice and encouragement, Enrica Ardemagni, PhD, Department of World Language and Cultures, Indiana University and Nataly Kelly of Common Sense Advisory; for expert help with the introductory text and cover design, (respectively) Bruce Merley and Eike Ten Kley of Pacific Interpreters; for the original layout design, Andrew Tonry; for her skillful proofreading, Dorothy Reed Roat; and for her unflagging cooperation during the design process, Danielle Mojonnier of Grinning Moon Creative; and finally to Cynthia Roat, without whom there would *be* no book, for her willingness to revisit these essays, sentence by sentence, to insure their accuracy, consistency and appropriateness for publication.

Gene Tonry
Pacific Interpreters

Table of Contents

Foreword

By Bruce T. Downing, PhD

This collection of essays on healthcare interpreting is a treasure-trove of practical information, advice, tricks of the trade, good sense and good humor, offered up by one of the true pioneers and experts in this exciting and growing field. We can all be grateful to Pacific Interpreters and author Cynthia E. Roat for sharing them with the rest of us.

I've had the honor of knowing Cindy Roat for more than 15 years. I've observed her as a trainer, discussion leader, discussant, and (though she would probably hate the word) orator—persuasively moving an audience. I've read many studies and reports she has written and even had the pleasure of working with her on research and writing. In everything she does, I see evidence of her common sense and breadth of knowledge, and the fruits of her rich and varied experience as a working interpreter.

This is an impressive set of carefully targeted, sound, and practical essays. The "bites" of wisdom offered here clearly reflect the writer's experience and good judgment. They include topics central to learning and practicing the art of healthcare interpreting, including some that formal training programs may omit—or fail to present in the immediately useful, down-to-earth way they are offered to us here. Fun and useful exercises round out the book.

Many interpreters have gotten their start in this work without access to the quality training that could help them make the most of their skills and avoid the many pitfalls interpreters face. The topics and tips found here will fill in gaps for these interpreters.

Others have received training, but will find that pointers from Cindy Roat will aid their understanding and add ideas and topics that may have gotten little attention in their training. And current students and their instructors will quickly recognize how the essays in this book serve to highlight, summarize, or supplement their lessons.

To quote the author's words (unit 34): "No matter how good we are as interpreters, we can always learn something more: vocabulary, interpreting skills, a new way of looking at our role, trends in the field, new technologies." The articles in this collection were clearly composed to support an interpreter's continuing professional education.

These essays will also benefit anyone who depends on interpreters to help them talk with folks who don't speak the same language, as well as anyone who supervises the work of interpreters. As interpreters are learning to do their work with increasing efficiency, accuracy, and professionalism, those who use their services—in person or over the phone —need to keep up, to be aware of good professional practices in interpreting, and to interact in ways that will ease the interpreter's job and create better rapport and information-sharing with patients.

Above all, every reader will enjoy Cindy Roat's uniquely lively, refreshing and engaging style. You can read the book through and top it all off with the crosswords and exercises in the final section. But here's my recommended dosage: a first "bite" to start your day and another as a bedtime snack, to refresh both mind and spirit.

Bruce Downing is Associate Professor of Linguistics and Director of the Program in Translation and Interpreting, College of Continuing Education, University of Minnesota.

Introduction

by Gene Tonry

If you are a healthcare interpreter, this book is for you. You might be part-time or full-time, interpreting on-site or over-the-phone, an employee or an independent contractor; whatever your connection to interpreting, we think you will find a wealth of useful information in this little book. If you are a student in an interpreter program (or would like to be), this book will give you a feel for what it is really like and you will receive lots of helpful guidance. If you are a dual-role interpreter (health care staff who is also trained as an interpreter), community interpreter, or volunteer, reading this book will leave you much better prepared. Finally, if your job includes communicating through interpreters or you simply work in a linguistically diverse environment, you will gain valuable understanding. To be sure, it is the environment of the future.

All of the articles in this book were written by Cynthia E. Roat for Pacific Interpreters' monthly communications vehicle to its interpreters, *The PI Newsletter*. Cindy (as she is known to interpreters, trainers and healthcare professionals throughout the U.S.) has been writing a monthly column for Pacific's Newsletter since 2001, and more than half of them are included here. Cindy is widely known for her contributions to interpreter training, consulting and research. She is the principal author of *Bridging the Gap*, the first widely-used training program for healthcare interpreters, and she has authored pioneering research papers which are standard references in the field. Her lively presentations are familiar to many who attend the annual conventions of the National Council on Interpreting in Health Care (NCIHC), the California Healthcare Interpreting Association (CHIA), the International Medical Interpreters Association

(IMIA), and similar organizations.

One of my responsibilities as a manager at Pacific Interpreters is overseeing the *Newsletter*. When I indexed the complete series of articles a year ago, I was struck by several things: first, the continuing relevance of Cindy's chosen topics; second, the empathy and regard for the interpreter's important role; and finally the approachability and often delightful sense of humor that, combined with impressive expertise, made the articles pleasurable reading.

I reference these articles again and again when answering questions from interpreters: questions like "How do I maintain professional boundaries without appearing unfriendly?" (See Chapter 3), "How do I interpret when there's no equivalent terminology in the other language?" (See Chapter 7), "Interpreting mental health encounters scares me. Can you give me some guidance?" (See Chapters 18-20), or "How do I handle an angry client?" (See Chapter 25).

The articles are arranged thematically. Section 1, "Tips and Tricks of the Trade," explains interpreting standards and protocols and includes tips on techniques such as improving memory, note-taking, and controlling the interpreting session. Section 2, "The Key to Success is Being Prepared," provides essential information for interpreting in pediatrics, the asthma clinic, pharmacy, genetic counseling, and behavioral health. It also addresses the challenges of sight translation and interpreting in end-of-life situations.

Section 3, "The Under-appreciated Interpreter," speaks candidly about the prejudice that every interpreter will encounter sooner or later (see Chapter 28, "Why Don't They Just Learn English?"), and gives advice on handling difficult situations.

Section 4, "Rx for Interpreters," addresses vocational and personal issues: the challenge of staying healthy while serving in health care (Chapter 29), and setting yourself up as a business (Chapter 30). This section includes "Interpreting with a Broken Heart," (Chapter 37), my personal favorite, which should not be missed.

The second part of the book contains exercises and crossword puzzles designed to review and expand medical vocabulary in English. Cindy dons her "Puzzle Mistress" cap and delves into a number of common interpreting situations, continuing the important theme of "Being Prepared" (Section 2) by another means. There are exercises on the terminology of obstetrics, nutrition, dentistry and cardiology; as well as a pair of exercises on the vocabulary of social services and a comprehensive review of "Idioms, Acronyms and Abbreviations."

In the 18+ years that Pacific Interpreters has provided interpreting services to the healthcare community we have taken great satisfaction in watching the profession grow and mature. Today there are dozens, perhaps even hundreds of professional training and educational programs that offer the healthcare interpreter many pathways for quality education and professional development. We even live on the eve of national certification for our interpreters! At the same time, the old "school of hard knocks" and "life in the trenches" still have so much wisdom and experience to offer to both the experienced and the aspiring medical interpreter. This wonderful little book of Cindy Roat's offerings "from the trenches" cannot but help enrich the skills, abilities and wisdom of all medical interpreters. Read, learn, savor and enjoy!

Part 1

Section 1

Tips and Tricks of the Trade

1.

There is No Egg in Eggplant
Coping with the English Language

Most interpreters have at least one thing in common with the people for whom we interpret: there was a time when we too spoke only one language. We, however, have learned at least one other. And for most healthcare interpreters in this country, one of those "others" was English.

As a native speaker of English, I would like to personally apologize to those of you who had to learn this language after childhood. I mean, really, could you invent a more difficult language, even if you tried? Just think about it! As an anonymous and much-quoted linguist has written:

> "There is no egg in eggplant or ham in hamburger; neither apple nor pine in pineapple. English muffins weren't invented in England nor French fries in France. Sweetmeats are candies while sweetbreads, which aren't sweet, are meat.
>
> " . . . quicksand can work slowly, boxing rings are square and a guinea pig is neither from Guinea nor is it a pig. And why is it that writers write but fingers don't fing, grocers don't groce and hammers don't ham? . . . Doesn't it seem crazy that you can make amends but not one amend, that you comb through annals of history but not a single annal? If you have a

> bunch of odds and ends and get rid of all but one of them, what do you call it? If teachers taught, why didn't preachers praught? If a vegetarian eats vegetables, what does a humanitarian eat?
>
> " . . . In what other language do people recite at a play and play at a recital? Ship by truck and send cargo by ship? Park on driveways and drive on parkways? Have noses that run and feet that smell? How can a slim chance and a fat chance be the same, while a wise man and a wise guy are opposites? You have to marvel at the unique lunacy of a language in which your house can burn up as it burns down, in which you fill in a form by filling it out and in which an alarm goes off by going on."[1]

But no, it's not true that English was developed specifically to torture those who try to learn it as a second language! English started out originally as Indo-European, an ancient language that branched into Romance (based on Latin), Germanic, Indo-Iranian, Slavic, Baltic and Celtic languages. English belongs to the Germanic group. It moved west out of mainland Europe with the Angles, Saxons and Jutes who invaded the British Isles in the fifth and sixth centuries A.D. But in 1066 A.D. William the Conqueror invaded England from Normandy, bringing with him Anglo-Norman, an early version of French. For centuries, then, the rulers of England spoke one language while the populace spoke another. Even today, one can see that many of the words commonly used by the aristocracy (such as "beef", which you eat) have their roots in French while the common man's vocabulary (such as "cow", which you take care of) remained more rooted in the Germanic English.

After England lost Normandy to the French in 1204 and the bubonic plague wiped out a third of the country's population in 1350, English rose in prominence over Anglo-Norman in England. The mixture of the two languages became Middle English, which flourished until the 16th century, when the Renaissance brought more Latinate words into the language. The printing press was introduced into England in 1476, leading to a process of standardization of grammar and spelling which was embodied in the publishing of the first English dictionary in 1604.

From the 1600's, the major changes in English have been in the addition of vocabulary. The industrial revolution initiated the need for a whole host of new words to describe things and processes previously unknown. This process continues today, especially in the world of technology. Secondly, the rise of the British Empire and global trade led to the introduction of English as a language of commerce and power around the world. It led as well to the introduction of words from many of the world's languages

[1]This article is posted all over the internet. However I have been unable to anywhere find an attribution. One posting of the entire article can be found at http://www.edu-cyberpg.com/Literacy/reading.asp

into English. In the U.S., in particular, the influence of Native American languages and Spanish has been significant.

So, no wonder English is a mess. The origins of the language in both Germanic and Anglo-Norman lead to a plethora of synonyms; almost everything has one word with a Germanic root and another with a Latinate root. The spelling and grammar were standardized four centuries ago, but pronunciation has continued to change. Then worldwide diffusion has led to enormous regional variations and a hodgepodge of vocabulary stolen from other languages! In fact, 99% of the words in the Oxford English Dictionary are borrowed from another language. This leads to rules for spelling and pronunciation for which there seem to be more exceptions than rules. Just consider:

1. The bandage was wound around the wound.
2. We produce produce on a farm.
3. A full dump must refuse refuse.
4. There is no time like the present to present a present.
5. Get the lead out and lead![2]

And that doesn't even count the words that are spelled differently but pronounced the same!

And yet, despite all this, English is a wildly popular language worldwide. Wikipedia, the on-line free encyclopedia, reports that English is the most widely taught and understood language in the world. Between 300 and 400 million people speak it as a first language, and The Times Online reports that about a third of the world's population (that's about a 1.9 billion people) has a basic proficiency in English. Certainly English has become the lingua franca in international trade, science, aviation, and the internet. English is chosen as a common language even in some international organizations in which no native English speakers participate, such as the European Central Bank.

And though English is not, as some people claim, the official language of the United States (the U.S. has no official language), it is certainly the language of common discourse here. That means that immigrants and refugees who weren't lucky enough to learn English before coming must learn it here if they want to advance economically and participate in the country's civil life. As we have seen, English is not an easy language to learn. Certainly the courtroom and the emergency room, where the potential consequences of misunderstanding can be very serious, are not the places to be practicing.

And that's where you come in. Interpreters bridge the language gap for non-English speakers seeking access to public services. You are the guide to this strange and

---

[2]Ibid

confusing language until the patient learns enough to get around the vernacular by himself. And, like any good guide, you must know your way through the complexities and seeming illogic of this language.

So to those of you who have already mastered English, congratulations! And for those who are still struggling with the language, no wonder! Don't give up, and if you get discouraged, just read this little ditty and you'll remember what you're up against. And what your patients are up against as well.

> We'll begin with a box, and the plural is boxes;
> But the plural of ox becomes oxen not oxes.
> One fowl is a goose, but two are called geese,
> Yet the plural of moose should never be meese.
> You may find a lone mouse or a nest full of mice;
> Yet the plural of house is houses, not hice.
> If the plural of man is always called men,
> Why shouldn't the plural of pan be called pen?
> The cow in a plural may be cows or kine,
> But the plural of vow is vows and not vine.
> If I speak of my foot and show you my feet,
> And I give you a boot, would a pair be called beet?
> If one is a tooth, and whole set are teeth,
> Why shouldn't the plural of booth be called beeth?
> Then one may be that, and three would be those,
> Yet hat in the plural would never be hose,
> And the plural of cat is cats, not cose.
> We speak of a brother and also of brethren,
> But though we say mother, we never say methren.
> Then the masculine pronouns are he, his and him,
> But imagine the feminine, she, shis and shim.
>
> - Alice Hess Beveridge
> (also attributed to Richard Ladere)

August 2006

2.

The Pre-session

The Interpreter's Magic Tool for Avoiding Frustration

"Patients don't seem to trust interpreters."
"Providers don't seem to trust interpreters."
"The patient and the doctor always talk to me, not to each other."
"Nobody pauses to let me interpret."
"Patients are always telling me things that they don't want interpreted."

Sound familiar? These are some of the most common frustrations that community interpreters run into. And though nothing you do will completely eradicate these problems, you do possess a tool that will minimize them: the pre-session.

What is a pre-session?

A pre-session is a short (sometimes very short) introduction that you do with the patient and provider before beginning the interpretation. The purposes of the pre-session are to introduce yourself, to establish yourself as a professional interpreter, to clarify your role, and to help patient and provider know how best to use your services. Remember, if a patient or provider has not worked previously with a professional interpreter, they won't know what to expect. You need to tell them.

How do I do a pre-session?

Pre-sessions with the patient can usually be done in a fairly relaxed manner, sitting next to the patient, since there is usually ample time. There is often time to do a pre-session with patients before the provider comes in, either while sitting in the waiting room, or while sitting in the exam room after the vital signs have been taken. Here are some things to include in a pre-session with a patient:

1. your name,
2. the organization you represent,
3. that the patient can speak directly to the provider,
4. that you'll interpret everything that is said exactly as it was said,
5. that it would help you be more accurate if he or she would pause after a full thought to let you interpret,
6. that all information will be kept confidential,
7. that you cannot answer questions or give medical advice.

Pre-sessions with the provider must be done more quickly, as they typically take place right after the provider comes in and introduces him- or herself to the patient. You will want to include many of the same things you told the patient:

1. your name,
2. the organization you represent,
3. that you'll interpret everything that is said exactly as it was said,
4. that the provider can speak directly to the patient,
5. that it would help you to be more accurate if he or she would pause after a full thought to let you interpret.

If you have worked before with a particular provider, you don't have to do a pre-session every time. However, if you've never done one before, do at least one with every patient and provider with whom you work!

So why don't interpreters do pre-sessions more often?

It's a mystery to me! As I train interpreters around the country, I find that many are reluctant to do pre-sessions. They tell me they are afraid it will take too much time, that the provider will be impatient, that it seems too formal with the patient. Yet when I train providers to work with interpreters and show them what a professional pre-session looks like, they say: "Wow, that's great! It really clarifies how things should work. I wish my interpreters would do that."

So, avoid the frustration of patients and providers who don't know how to work with you. Do everyone a favor, and do a pre-session.

March, 2002

3.

The Art of Being Polite

I remember the first business letter I ever received in Spanish. Written by a colleague at the Ministry of Health in Ecuador, it started out something like this:

> *"A través de la presente, reciba Ud. un muy cordial saludo de parte de su servidor, junto con la esperanza de que la presente la encuentre gozando de buena salud y rodeada por los suyos."*

Or, literally:

> "By means of this letter, may you receive a very warm greeting from your servant, together with the hope that this letter finds you enjoying good health and surrounded by your loved ones."

Having grown up in a country where a business letter should get to the point in the first three words, I remember thinking that this was a silly way to begin and wondering why this colleague was writing in such a ridiculously formal fashion. (OK, so I was young and culturally incompetent!) After living in Ecuador for a while, however, I began to appreciate how gracious this fashion was, how respectful -- and how widespread. This was not some flowery poetry that this colleague had composed for me; it was a standard, polite way to start a business letter.

Every language has such constructs. There are polite ways to greet someone, to ask for a favor, to interrupt, to apologize. They can't be changed; the words have to be just so. Sometimes we learn these constructs when we learn a second language, but often we don't. As a result, while we may do fine in everyday conversation, we seem rude, uneducated or boorish in certain situations. I can't imagine what my Ecuadorian colleagues thought of my business letters before someone taught me the "formulas!"

So, why am I writing about this in an interpreting bulletin? As interpreters, we spend most of our time in the background, repeating in one language a message that was expressed in another. At times, however, we need to speak for ourselves. We need to intervene, ask for a repeat, point out a potential misunderstanding, ask for clarification. If we have not learned the polite formulas in English, we - and the company for which we work - can look very unprofessional.

So, here are some of the formulas used in English that will mark you as an educated, polite, respectful and professional interpreter. Tape them to your bathroom mirror and practice a few every day. Clients and friends will be suitably impressed!

When introduced:

> "Ms. A, this is Mr. B."
> "Pleased to meet you." Or "A pleasure."
> And the proper response is: "The pleasure is mine."

When intervening to ask for repetition:

> "The interpreter asks if you could please repeat your last sentence." or
> "The interpreter would like to request a repeat."

When intervening to ask for clarification:

> "Speaking as the interpreter, could you please explain to me what you meant by ____________?"

When intervening to check for understanding:

> "As the interpreter, I am concerned that Ms. X did not understand how she is to take her medication. Would it be acceptable for me to ask?"

When intervening in the role of culture broker (for example):

> "I couldn't take this medication, because it's too hot. The interpreter says, the way the patient is using this word "hot" has a special meaning in his culture. Would it be helpful to you if I explained it?"

When bringing up a problem:

"I am concerned. . . ."

When suggesting a solution

"I was wondering if .. ."

When forced to interrupt:

"Forgive me for interrupting."

When thanking someone:

"I very much appreciate your help. . ." or
"You are very kind."

And a polite response when thanked:

"It was my pleasure." or
"Think nothing of it." or
"Consider me at your disposal."

Here are some other tips that will mark you as a polite and professional interpreter.

- Avoid blaming. Professionals focus first on how to solve a problem, not on who caused it.
- Disagree, but don't contradict.
- Try not to interrupt unless absolutely necessary.
- Be slow to judge and quick to apologize.
- Start statements or questions with "I" instead of "you". For example, instead of saying "You never said that!" you could say, "I didn't hear you say that."
- Always stay calm. In the dominant culture here, professional people do not raise their voices at each other. Get mad when you hang up, but while on the line, don't lose your cool.

Sociologists tell us that up to 70% of a message is not in the words, but in how the words are said. Learning these tips, and choosing your words and tone of voice carefully, will assure that you will always be perceived as the professional you are and be welcomed wherever you go.

February, 2003

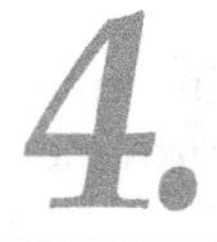

Transparency Means Clarity

Using Intervention Skills to Keep Communication on Track

Ask providers what behavior most rapidly erodes their trust in an interpreter, and chances are they'll cite one of two situations:

1. When the interpretation is a lot longer or a lot shorter than the original speech.
2. When the interpreter gets into a conversation with the patient that excludes the provider.

If you ask the the patient, you're likely to hear the same.

As interpreters, we understand what everyone around us is saying. It is terribly tempting in an interpreted session to use our own voices to "make things better:" to sooth a patient's fears, to chat with a doctor or nurse, to redirect a patient who's not answering the doctor's question, to cut off a rambling story, to respond to a question whose answer you know. You may think that by talking to the patient or provider directly you are saving the provider time.

But from the point of view of the monolingual, there is something naturally unsettling about listening to two people converse in a language you don't understand when you are supposed to be part of the conversation. As patients and providers get more accustomed to working with professional interpreters, they have come to expect, quite justifiably, that everything that is said will be interpreted and that interpreters will stay in the background. There is a good reason for this; everything a patient or provider says carries information to the listener about health history, symptoms, attitudes, diagnosis, or directions. All of this is important in developing a relationship and in diagnosing and treating the patient's health problems. Any speech that is not interpreted robs the provider or the patient of that potentially crucial information and distracts the focus of the conversation away from the patient-provider dialogue.

In addition, many providers have suffered through enough unprofessional interpreting that they have become highly sensitive to the possibility that interpreters may be interjecting their opinions of what is being said, giving advice to patients, or adding information that could be clinically incorrect. If you are trying to lose the trust of a provider, talking to the patient without provider knowing what's happening would be just the way to do it.

So, the general lesson for interpreters is: just interpret. Don't make comments, don't ask questions, don't get into conversations directly with the patient (or the provider, for that matter). Just interpret.

But wait a minute - aren't there times when an interpreter has a valid reason to intervene in the conversation? Aren't there times when an interpreter must stop to ask a question or help clarify a confusion? Yes, there certainly are.

As interpreters, we intervene for a variety of good reasons: we didn't understand what was just said; we think the patient didn't understand what we just interpreted; a cultural issue has come up; we need a repeat; we need someone to pause more often. There are others. So, what do you do if you have a valid reason to intervene, but you don't want to lose the provider's trust? The key is being transparent.

Being transparent means that, if you have a valid reason to talk to just one party in an encounter, you tell the other party what you are going to do first. The technique requires some practice, but once you get the hang of it, your interventions can be smooth, effective and quickly over.

The steps for intervention are

1. Interpret as much of what the speaker said as you can.
2. Tell the listener what you need to ask or do.
3. Ask the speaker your question or share the information you need to share.

4. Go back to interpreting.

Here are some examples:

Example A. You don't understand what the patient just said and you need her to explain it.

> *"The baby wouldn't stop crying and so I gave mumble, mumble, mumble."*
>
> 1. Interpret what you did understand to the provider first:
>
> "The baby wouldn't stop crying and so I gave ---"
>
> 2. Tell the provider that you need the patient to explain the rest:
>
> "The interpreter says, I need her to clarify the last part of what she said."
>
> 3. Ask the patient to explain to you:
>
> *"As the interpreter, I'm asking, could you repeat what you said?"*
>
> 4. Once you understand, go back to interpreting:
>
> "I couldn't get the baby to stop crying, so I gave her a bottle with chamomile tea."

Example B. You've been interpreting accurately, but the patient is not responding. You think the patient didn't understand, and you want to check.

> "Because of your age and parity, you fall into a population considered at high risk to produce a fetus with a chromosomal disorder like Down Syndrome."
>
> 1. Interpret what the provider said to the patient first:
>
> "Because of your age and parity, you fall into a population considered at high risk to produce a fetus with a chromosomal disorder like Down Syndrome."
>
> 2. Tell the provider that you are concerned that the patient is not understanding and you would like to check:
>
> *"As the interpreter, I'm concerned that the patient is not understanding. May I ask what she understood of what you just said?"*
>
> 3. Ask the patient what she understood:

"As the interpreter, I wanted to ask what you understood of what the counselor just told you."

4. Interpret the patient's answer to the physician and go back to interpreting:

"I don't know, I didn't understand what she said."

Example C. The provider is using technical terminology that you don't understand.

"Have you ever been diagnosed with ketoacidosis?"

1. Interpret what you did understand to the patient:

"Have you ever been diagnosed with --- "

2. Add that you need clarification of the rest:

"As the interpreter, I need to ask the doctor what he meant."

3. Ask the provider for clarification:

"The interpreter needs clarification of ketoacidosis."

4. Interpret the response to the patient and go back to interpreting:

"Have you ever been diagnosed with a very high blood sugar level and high levels of ketones in your blood and urine?

Being transparent, then, assures that everyone in the conversation knows what is being said. No information is lost and trust is maintained. Transparency is a sure way to avoid that second most common complaint that providers have with interpreters. So be transparent. Be clear. Be professional.

August, 2009

5.

In the Language of Interpreters, How Do You Say "Helpful?"

Understanding the Role of the Interpreter

Rumor has it that some of you interpreters out there are being helpful to patients and providers. That's great! Or rather, I mean, that's terrible!

Wait a minute. Is it great or is it terrible? I guess it depends on what we mean by "helpful." How *do* you say "helpful" in the language of interpreters?

The answer is to be found in definition of the interpreter's role. Why are we there? What is the purpose of the interpreter? One common definition is this:

> "The purpose of the interpreter is to facilitate understanding in communication between people speaking different languages."[3]

So, being helpful as an interpreter means taking away the language barrier and allowing two people who don't speak the same language to understand each other. Is our purpose to improve on what someone said, make it nicer, make it more what the listener expects? No, we're not responsible for WHAT is said, only for making sure it

[3]Roat, Cynthia. *Bridging the Gap: A Basic Training for Medical Interpreters.* The Cross Cultural Health Care Program, 1999.

was understood. Is our purpose to explain medical concepts? Negative; that's what the health care provider is trained to do. Is it our purpose to find out the answers to the social worker's questions? Uh-uh; that's the social worker's job; ours is to make sure the patient understood the social worker's questions. Is our purpose to be everyone's friend? Nope: friendly, but not friends. We are polite and professional, and so we help build trust between the patient and the provider. We stay in the background.

Changing what was said, adding to what was said, leaving out parts of what was said, jumping ahead to what we think might be said next - this is not being helpful as an interpreter. When we do these things, we are taking over the role and the work of the provider, the social worker, or the patient - whoever the speaker is. While we may think we are being helpful, we are really being disrespectful, undercutting each speaker's right to speak for him or herself. Being helpful as an interpreter means reproducing faithfully in one language the meaning that was expressed in another. The more accurately and completely you can do that, the more helpful you are being.

Now, somebody out there must be protesting, "But the nurse asks me to find out all the vaccinations the child has. If I just interpret her question to the patient, I won't get all the information, and I haven't done a good job." Actually, if you interpret the nurse's question, you have done a great job -- as an interpreter. You haven't done a very good job as a nurse. But you aren't a nurse; you're an interpreter. Let the nurse ask the questions; you interpret. If the nurse complains that you weren't "helpful", explain to her how a professional interpreter works. More likely, as providers learn more about how to work with interpreters, the provider will commend you when you stay in your role and help by removing the language barrier.

A test!

So, here's a little test for you. Read each statement of behavior below and put a ☆ after it if it is an example of how a professional interpreter is helpful. Put a ⦸ after it, if it is an example of how an interpreter is NOT really being helpful. Then check page 27 to see how you did! And go out there and be HELPFUL today, as only a truly professional interpreter can be.

1. The patient's reply doesn't seem to answer the doctor's question. You interpret exactly what the patient said. The provider seems a bit annoyed, and then asks the question in a different way. ______
2. The patient is being seen for chronic stomach pain. When the doctor asks about how long it has hurt, the patient says about one month, and then starts to tell the doctor about how worried she is about her son. You break in and interpret "One month," saving the doctor from having to listen to a long story that has nothing to do with the doctor's question. ______

3. You are getting to the end of what you can remember as the patient speaks. The patient pauses for a second or two, so you slip in and start to interpret. ______
4. The patient is really angry about how he has been treated. To smooth things out, you interpret what he has said into much softer, politer language. ______
5. You are interpreting over the phone, and the patient's story is very sad. She seems lonely, as if she really needs a friend. While the doctor puts you on hold, you talk to the patient, try to cheer her up and give her your home phone number so she can call you if she needs someone to talk to. ______
6. The surgical scheduler has called a patient to tell her that he cannot schedule her surgery because she has not sent in the appropriate referral. The patient says the doctor said for her to have the surgery. The conversation goes around and around, with each side getting more and more frustrated. You start to suspect that the patient may not understand the word "referral," since there is no exact equivalent for this term in the patient's language. You say to the scheduler, "As the interpreter, I'd like to ask the patient how she understood my interpretation of "referral," since this term doesn't exist in her language." ______
7. The patient's answer didn't really answer the provider's question. So you try again, asking the question in a different way. You have to ask three or four times, but you finally get a straight answer out of the patient. ______
8. The doctor on the phone says to you, "Find out what's wrong with him." You reply, "Speaking as the interpreter, if you could talk directly to the patient as you would an English-speaking patient, I'll interpret exactly what you say." ______
9. You are interpreting on the phone for financial services. You've interpreted for dozens of these calls, and they are all the same. So, to save time for the client, you anticipate the next two or three questions. This way, you can report back the answers before the financial services representative even has to ask the questions. ______
10. The patient is calling in with an emergency. The patient is very upset, but the provider taking the call seems totally unaffected, calm and detached. You feel like the provider isn't very empathetic, and the patient seems upset by the provider's attitude. You think that if you could tell the patient that you understand what she is going through, you could improve her rapport with the provider. But you limit yourself to just interpreting what is being said. ______

11. The patient has just answered a question about his income in such a way that you know will make him ineligible for the help he is requesting. You realize he probably has no idea that what he has said will make him ineligible, so you change it a little to help him out. ______
12. You are interpreting for a triage session with a consulting nurse. This is the fourth time this week someone has called in with virtually the same type of respiratory symptoms. Every other time, the nurse has told the patient, among other things, to take aspirin for the fever. This time, she didn't mention the aspirin. Since this is clearly an oversight on her part, and since the patient seems to have the same thing as the other patients on the other calls, you let the patient know to take aspirin for the fever. ______

June 2002

Answers

1. ☆

2. ⃠

3. ☆

4. ⃠

5. ⃠

6. ☆

7. ☆

8. ☆

9. ⃠

10. ☆

11. ⃠

12. ⃠

6.

Confidentiality Across Cultures

> "The interpreter treats as confidential, within the treating team, all information learned in the performance of their professional duties, while observing relevant requirements regarding disclosure."
>
> From A National Code of Ethics for Interpreters in Health Care,
> The National Council on Interpreting in Health Care, 2004.

If you've heard it once, you've heard it a thousand times: interpreters maintain confidentiality at all times. It is one of the hallmarks of a professional interpreter and one of the most important keys to establishing our credibility with both providers and patients. We sign confidentiality agreements with hospitals. We assure patients in the pre-sessions that we will keep all information secret. We destroy interpreting notes to safeguard confidentiality.

But have you ever wondered if you, the hospital and the patient all understand the same thing when you promise to "treat as confidential . . . all information learned in the performance of (your) professional duties?" A quick survey of professional medical interpreters suggests that we all may not share the same definition of this key concept.

This should not surprise us. As you know, culture impacts how we interpret and interact with the world. It is not strange, then, that people from different cultures should interpret a sensitive word like "confidential" in different ways. Let's look at some of those distinctions.

Here's how the Merriam-Webster dictionary defines "confidential:"

> **con•fi•den•tial**
> Pronunciation: kän-fi-'den(t)-shel
> Function: adjective
> 1 : marked by intimacy or willingness to confide, "a confidential tone"
> 2 : private, secret "confidential information"
> 3 : entrusted with confidences , "confidential clerk"
> 4 : containing information whose unauthorized disclosure could be prejudicial to the national interest - compare secret, top secret

In the dominant culture in this country, "confidential" is generally understood to mean "secret." When a friend tells you something "in confidence," she is expecting that you won't tell anyone. Period. We often think of "confidential" as being like the status of confessions to a priest, which he may not divulge to anyone under any circumstances at all.

Medical culture, on the other hand, has a slightly different understanding of "confidential." Personal information is kept confidential in that only the people who need to know that information are party to it. However that can include everyone from the receptionist to the medical assistant to the nurse to the doctor to the phlebotomist to the interpreter to the billing clerk. Sometimes it can seem that your secret is not much of a secret in a health care institution.

For interpreters, the meaning of "confidential" has changed over the past decade. It used to mean "secret" — sort of. Professional spoken-language interpreters did not repeat what they had heard in interpreted sessions, except in cases of mandated reporting or for educational purposes (without revealing identifiers). The Code of Ethics of the Registry of Interpreters for the Deaf used to be so strict on this issue that it didn't allow interpreters to tell anyone that they were even going to an interpreting assignment. Now, however the revised RID Code is more realistic, focusing on prohibiting gossip instead of constituting a gag order. And the National Code of Ethics for Interpreters in Health Care, published by the National Council on Interpreting in Health Care, has adopted the meaning of "confidentiality" prevalent in health care in general and described above.

How do LEP patients understand "confidentiality?" That depends, of course on both the patient's cultural roots and the patient's personal culture. But here are some suggestions shared by working interpreters on the listserv of the National Council on Interpreting in Health Care, of the different ways in which they have seen this word applied.

One Russian-English interpreter writes that she has noticed, and confirmed with recently immigrated Russian physicians, that her patients understand "confidentiality" to mean that sensitive information is never divulged to the **patient** nor to anyone untrustworthy enough to tell the patient. The patient must be protected from bad news. Clearly this differs significantly from what U.S. health systems have in mind.

Another Russian-English interpreter reports that her Russian colleagues and family understand "confidentiality" as does the dominant culture here. She mentions that other Russians, though, commonly understand that all "confidential" information will be passed as a matter of course to the patient's close family. In this country, that would be considered a clear breach of confidentiality.

Maria Carr, a Spanish-English interpreter, writes that after years of medical interpreting, she has come to the conclusion that the concept of confidentiality as it is used in the U.S. health care system does not exist for many Spanish-speaking patients. Assurances that information will be kept confidential are met with blank stares and confused looks. The word "confidential" must be explained. She goes on to explain why she thinks this may be so:

> "My personal experience growing up in a Mexican culture at home taught me that families, neighbors, friends and even acquaintances have a genuine interest in and concern for each other. Therefore, any time someone is hurt, sick, having a baby, lost a loved one, etc., they are surrounded by a group of concerned and loving people from all those groups. The idea of showing support for each other also seems to be closely related to the idea of respect. It is a sign of respect to show up in support of those enjoying or suffering through life's ups and downs. The recipient of this support doesn't seem to be the least concerned that everyone knows the particulars of what's going on in their life. Instead I have experienced (in my own family too) almost a sense of obligation (again from respect/ social courtesy) to receive all the well-wishers and allow them even a brief visit to offer congratulations, best wishes, sympathy, prayers, etc."
>
> — Maria Carr, personal correspondence, November 29, 2005
> (Reproduced with permission)

So in Maria's point of view, her Spanish-speaking patients may seem confused by the concern about keeping everything secret, because telling appropriate people so that those people can be supportive is considered a kindness.

I found a similar point of view when training Hmong interpreters in Montana. These interpreters happened to be clan leaders in their communities. When we discussed the requirements to maintain confidentiality, they were chagrined. It was their role in the community, they explained, to let people know what was happening to a patient so that the community could offer appropriate support. The patient could not tell anyone, as that would be considered immodest. It was the clan leader's role to do so. In their eyes, the stricture to keep everything confidential was cruel and isolated the patient from his/her support systems.

Russian Pentecostal interpreters in this same training insisted that confidentiality was unnecessary in their interpreting because nobody in their community had anything they would want kept secret from each other. Interestingly enough, the one non-Pentecostal Russian interpreter in town told me that she was often specifically requested expressly because the patient wanted to discuss something with the doctor that he or she knew would be criticized in the community.

Indeed, it is not unusual for patients in small cultural communities to choose to use telephonic interpreters for particular medical visits specifically because those interpreters, commonly situated outside the geographic community, cannot share any information with the local community. Perhaps these patients welcome sharing information about health problems for which there will be community support but prefer confidentiality when the problem is one that carries a social stigma.

What can we conclude from all this, then? We need to start by realizing that the word "confidentiality" is not understood the same by all who hear it. As interpreters, we need to understand and apply confidentiality as it is understood and applied by the health care team of which we are a part. When we mention it to patients, however, we may need to explain more fully what we mean, or use a paraphrase to describe the concept. Differing cultures will lead to differing expectations among patients about what this word means. By explaining more clearly, we can both clarify what we mean in the moment and avoid culturally based confusions later on.

And that's not something that should be kept secret by any of us.

December, 2005

When There is No Word for That

Compensation Strategies for Interpreters

> "Your advocate at the shelter is going to help you qualify for Section 8 Housing. Meanwhile, we'd like you to join a support group for abused women, to work on your self-esteem. If you can open up to someone there and process some of your trauma, it'll help you get more centered."

Whoa! "advocate," "shelter," "Section 8 housing," "support group," "self-esteem" - how can you possibly interpret this? Half of the words and concepts simply have no equivalent in many target languages. Compensating for this discrepancy is a high level skill that interpreters continue to develop throughout their careers, first by realizing when a compensation strategy is necessary and then by deciding which to use.

When do you need to employ a compensation strategy? There are two general situations:

1. When no linguistic (or sometime conceptual) equivalent exists. For example, many languages have no words for mental health, privacy, self-esteem, down-time, time-out. They may not even have the idea. The same is true of English: the Asian concept of "hot and cold" does not exist in English, nor does an equivalent concept for the idea of *chi*.

2. When a linguistic equivalent doesn't carry the same meaning. Even more often, a linguistic equivalent could be constructed, but it won't mean the same thing. For example, you might be able to find words that seem to be the literal equivalent to English terms such as "advocate," "shelter," "red flag," "Section 8 Housing." But they wouldn't convey the same meaning in the target language. The same is often true of acronyms, such as TANF, DSHS, SSI, WIC, and of culturally based references.

How often these situations arise when you interpret depends largely on your language pair and to some degree on your listener. Interpreters of English and Cambodian, two very dissimilar languages spoken by members of very different cultures, have a bigger challenge than interpreters of English and Spanish, two languages that share more linguistic and conceptual equivalence. Speakers and listeners with a higher degree of common experience with a topic of conversation will need the interpreter to use fewer compensation strategies.

So, how do you deal with this lack of equivalence? First of all, remember that you are interpreting meaning, not words. In many cases, this will solve the problem. For example, let's say that a doctor is explaining to a mother when to bring her baby back to the ER. He tells her that "the following are red flags." If you focus on interpreting words, you're in trouble. If you interpret meaning though, it should be easy to find a term that means "warning signs," "signs of trouble," "signs of danger" or something similar.

But what if there isn't any easy equivalent to the meaning or a word or phrase? Consider the word "advocate." This is a term that describes a role that does not exist, or isn't named as such, in many cultures. Now what? You have two choices: you can ask the speaker to explain the term, or you can build a word picture of the meaning.

Asking for an explanation is a skill in itself. You need to be transparent in your question, be clear about what you want explained, make sure the rest of the utterance doesn't get lost and get back to interpreting as quickly as possible. Here's an example:

Social Worker (in English): "You might qualify for Section 8 Housing."

Interpreter (in the non-English language): *"You might qualify for 'Section 8 Housing.' As the interpreter, I'm going to ask for an explanation of Section 8 Housing."*

Interpreter to the Social Worker (in English): "The interpreter needs an explanation of the phrase 'Section 8 Housing.'"

Social Worker: "Section 8 Housing is rental housing that is subsidized by the government."

Interpreter (in the non-English language): *"Section 8 Housing is made up of houses and apartments for which the government helps pay part of the rent."*

Asking for clarification has the benefit of making the speaker define his or her own terms so you don't have to. However, as you can see, this can get very cumbersome if there are many terms that lack equivalence in the same sentence. In these cases, **if you know the meaning of the term**, it is more useful to build a word picture.

A good word picture has the following characteristics:

- It uses a definition form.
  For example, "Self-esteem means. . ."

- It is accurate.
  For example, a description of Section 8 Housing as a program in which the government pays for your house is not accurate. Under Section 8, the government helps pay rent on certain properties. The difference is important.

- It is precise.
  Vague descriptions are not useful. For example, a description of Section 8 Housing simply as a government program may be accurate, but it doesn't have enough details for the listener to really understand what it means within the conversation.

- It is efficient.
  Too much detail is confusing, though, and gets the interpretation off track. The trick to building word pictures is to include enough detail to be clear, but no more. Considering that, which is the better word picture of "food stamps"?

  "The card you use in the supermarket; the government puts money in its account; you'll get it from your case manager at the Senior Services Agency and then you can use it at the store to pay for food until all the money in the account is used up, which is usually the end of the month."

  OR

  "A plastic card from the government that allows you to buy food at certain grocery stores."

> Obviously, the second version communicates the meaning clearly without adding unnecessary or confusing detail, and is a much better choice.

So, using these techniques, let's try to do a paraphrase of that first paragraph, assuming that the terms "advocate," "shelter", "Section 8 Housing," support group," "abused," "self-esteem," "open up," "trauma" and "centered" have no easily-understood equivalents in our target language.

> "The person assigned to help you at the safe house where you are staying is going to help you get into a special house or apartment for which the government pays some of the rent. Meanwhile, we'd like you to come to meetings with a group of women who get together to talk to and help each other. All these women have been beaten by someone they were living with. Talking to other women with your same experiences will help you feel better about yourself. If you can talk to other people about the bad things that have happened to you, it will help you feel peace inside."

To summarize, remember that we always interpret **meaning, not words.** If there is an equivalent term in your target language to the one used by the speaker, use it. If not, ask the speaker to clarify, or build a word picture of your own - one that is accurate, precise and efficient. Happy interpreting!

July 2003/May 2009

8.

Some Notes on Note-taking for Telephone Interpreters

I received a note the other day, noting that telephone interpreters might find useful an article on taking notes. This struck a note with me, because note-taking is certainly a noteworthy topic, especially for telephonic interpreters who (you've probably note-iced) tend to take notably more notes than on-site health care interpreters. So, I made a note to myself to write this article on note-taking.

Let me start by saying that I am by no means a pro at note-taking as an interpreter. However, I have received a few tips from some "noted" experts, and here they are. Try them out and let me know how they worked for you.

And on that note --- let's start with why you might want to improve your note-taking skills.

Experts suggest that there are four situations in which any interpreter should take careful notes:

1. When interpreting about a subject with which you are unfamiliar.
   If you are interpreting for a financial intake for the 357th time, you probably don't need notes at all; you probably have the questions and typical responses memorized. On the other hand, if you are

suddenly faced with a call in a medical specialty you've never heard of, you better get that pencil out.

2. When direct quotes are used.
   This doesn't happen too much in health care interpreting, but there may be some things said that you need to reproduce verbatim.

3. When interpreting numbers, names and lists of anything over three.
   These are the hardest to remember, so it's better to take notes than to make an error.

4. When you are tired.
   Interpreting is exhausting work. If you find yourself going blank, searching for words, interpreting from English into English (it happens to all of us on occasion!), this is a sign that your mind is getting tired. If you can take a break, do so. If not, take better notes.

Telephone interpreters in particular need to be able to take good notes. It's harder to control the flow of the dialogue over the phone than it is in person, so you may have more "run-on" speakers than you would if you were present for the interpreted encounter. An on-site interpreter can use a hand signal or other non-verbal communication to get a speaker to pause, but a telephone interpreter has fewer options. If the old "jump-in-when-they-take-a-breath" technique doesn't work, taking good notes is your next best bet.

Another reason to take good notes is that speakers on telephone encounters have a harder time getting the idea that they're talking with each other, not to you. As a result, speakers tend to ask multiple questions or give multiple directions at once, much more than you would find when interpreting on site. Your only hope? Good notes.

How complete your notes need to be depends on the particular session. In sessions in which speakers are pausing often, and the subject matter is quite familiar to you, you may take only cursory notes, jotting down (for example) only names, numbers, and addresses.

If the speakers in the session are running on without pausing, or if you are unfamiliar with the matter being discussed, you will need to take more complete notes (unless you've got one doozy of a good memory). Here are three major principles in note-taking for interpreters.

First of all, keep in mind that your notes are only there to jog your memory. You are not writing a transcript; you want to write just enough to remind yourself of what was said. Because of this, you do not want to use secretarial shorthand. This was a technique designed to record every word, and that is not the purpose of interpreter note-taking.

Secondly, you should be analyzing and understanding the speech as you are taking notes. Commit to memory the main lines of reasoning – the "big picture," so to speak. Then take notes on the details or the logical linkages. Your notes then complement what you remember of the general gist of the speech.

Interpreter notes consist of symbols, not whole words. You don't have time to write whole words. Using symbols instead of words is not only faster; it allows you to read directly from your notes into the target language. There is no single set of symbols that everyone uses; you need to make up your own. After all, they only need to make sense to you. Keep the symbols simple and few. Master note-takers use 50-120 ideograms at most, written with the fewest strokes possible.

Here are some examples of symbols that some interpreters use in note-taking. Remember, the symbols have to make sense to you. Notice how some symbols can build on others.

today	t	signs / symptoms	ss
tomorrow	t•	exam / test	x
yesterday	•t	blood test	bx
next week	w•	urine test	ux
last week	•w	fasting	npo
next month	m•	prescription	Rx
last month	•m	over the counter	otc
three weeks ago	•3w	beginning / start	∂
three weeks from now	3w•	end / stop	Ω
lower / go down /less	▼	pain	!
increase /go up / more	▲	dizziness	≈
not sure	?	nausea and vomiting	n/v

Of course, as you have no doubt realized, using a system like this requires that you take the time to develop and practice the use of your symbols. Don't try to invent symbols on the fly. Develop them, record them, and practice them, over and over again until their use is second nature.

In terms of technique, take notes on a narrow pad (3-4 inches only) or draw a line down the middle of a regular 8½" x 11" sheet of paper. Leave a small margin on the left. Take your notes horizontally, but start a new line for every new idea. Remember to keep your ideograms simple. If you have trouble at the end interpreting from your notes, take fewer notes and commit more to memory.

Finally, make sure you destroy those notes at the conclusions of the session. Even though only you can read them, the requirements of confidentiality demand that any notes about the patient be put in the patient's chart or destroyed. Make it a habit, and you'll never have to think about it twice.

And on that note, I'll close. Just remember, when you get ready to interpret over the phone, make sure you have a pad of paper and a pen or pencil close at hand. In terms of the quality of your interpreting, you'll find it will make a "noticeable" difference.

December 2002

9.

Memory Techniques for Healthcare Interpreters

Now just where did I put my notes for this article . . . h'm, did I put them . . . nope . . . I thought they were . . . not there either. I wish I could remember . . . Aha! Here they are! Right in this file of things I am supposed to remember to do . . .

You know, I really should try to improve my memory, because a good memory is critical for interpreters, especially those who do dialogue consecutive interpreting. In addition to just plain old good recall, though, there are many tricks that interpreters use in order to remember and reproduce a spoken message accurately. Here are a few.

1. Concentrate.

Interpreting takes a great deal of cognitive effort. Most of us just can't do it well if we are distracted, thinking about something else, upset, or mentally engaged elsewhere. Like any other creative activity, interpreting requires total concentration. To achieve this level of concentration, practice the following.

Sit in a chair with your back against the backrest. Cross your hands in your lap. Avert your gaze from making eye contact with anyone. Take a deep breath. Clear your mind of any worries you have, of thoughts about what you have done that day or will do later. Tune out background noise. Focus exclusively on what is being said, and (if you are interpreting in-person) on the body language of the speakers.

This complete concentration allows your mind to dedicate itself entirely to remembering a message and converting it to another language.

2. Visualize the action.

One the most useful memory techniques that I have found is visualization. This is especially useful when patients are telling their symptoms or the story of their illness, injury or prior treatment. As they describe what happened, imagine it as a video, playing in your mind. When you start to interpret, it will be easy to "rewind" the video and describe the same series of events in the target language.

3. Clump meaning and echo key words.

Clearly, we don't need to remember the exact words a speaker said; we need to remember and interpret the exact **meaning** of what was said. So all we really have to remember are key "trigger" words that will bring up in our minds the full meaning to be interpreted. For example, a doctor says "OK, you'll need to go down to radiology and have a X-ray taken. Bring back the film, give it to the receptionist, and I'll take a look at it. Then we'll decide how to proceed." In this 35-word utterance, there are really only 5 ideas, and each could be remembered by a one-word "trigger":

- Go to radiology – "radiology"
- Get an x-ray – "x-ray"
- Come back – "back"
- Give the film to the receptionist – "receptionist"
- Then we'll decide what to do – "decide"

If you can remember the concepts of "radiology", "x-ray", "back", "receptionist" and "decide," your memory will be triggered and your mind will fill in the rest of the words all by itself.

4. Count lists.

In health care interpreting, we often are asked to interpret lists: list of illnesses, lists of medicines, lists of instructions. Counting off (even on your fingers), the number of items in a list will actually help you remember them, or at the very least, to realize if you've left something out. So, when the nurse asks "Have you ever had diabetes, heart trouble, glaucoma, or a stroke?" get those fingers ready!

5. Take notes.

Telephone interpreters tend to take more notes than on-site interpreters, partially because speakers tend to run-on more over the phone, but also because it is more difficult to control the flow over the phone and easier to take notes sitting at a desk without anyone watching. Note-taking techniques are the subject of a separate article. However, you may be surprised how much you can remember without taking notes.

Memory Exercise

The key to internalizing the techniques listed above is practice. Here's an exercise you can do at home to help practice these skills.

Instructions

Before you start, compose yourself and empty your mind of other thoughts. Focus only on what you are going to hear. Choose a technique you want to practice: visualization of what is happening, clumping meaning and echoing the important words, counting key points or taking notes. Then have someone read you this story. Then, using your technique of choice, repeat the story back to your reader. Ask the reader to check off each key point that you remember.

The Story

My son was playing at the playground this afternoon with his friend Jessie. Jessie's is bigger than my son - about 7 years old. They were all over the place - the swings, the slide, the monkey bars, the merry-go-round. I was watching them and talking with my friend Grace who was there with me. They were just out of sight for a minute! Then suddenly, my son was running toward me, crying. I didn't even see it happen, but I figured he fell off the monkey bars. Then I realized that he was yelling Jessie's name, and I ran to where Jessie was lying on the ground. He was unconscious, but I know he was breathing - I checked that. I was scared to move him, so that's when I called 911."

Rating

Now rate yourself. Give yourself one point if you mentioned that:

1. Your son was playing at the playground.
2. You son's friend was there too.
3. Your son's friend is named Jessie.
4. The friend is older.
5. The friend is 7 years old.
6. The two boys were playing on many different pieces of equipment.
7. They were playing on the swings.

8. They were playing on the slide.
9. They were playing on the monkey bars.
10. They were playing on the merry-go-round.
11. You were watching the kids play.
12. You were talking with your friend.
13. Your friend's name is Grace.
14. The boys were out of sight for a minute.
15. Your son came running toward you.
16. Your son was crying.
17. You didn't see what happened.
18. You thought he might have fallen off the monkey bars.
19. Your son was yelling Jessie's name.
20. Jessie was lying on the ground.
21. Jessie was unconscious.
22. Jessie was breathing
23. You checked the breathing.
24. You didn't want to move him.
25. You called 911.

How did you do? Make up another story and try again. As simple as it may seem, this sort of practice is what will help you internalize these skills to the point that they will come to you without thinking when you start an interpreted session.

Memory skills and terminology are two areas that professional interpreters never stop working on. The better your memory skills, the smoother the interpreted session will go. So get to it; start practicing!

That is, if you can remember where you left the print-out of this article . . .

December 2003

10.

Interpreter as Advocate – Yes or No?

Few topics inspire such passionate debate among working health care interpreters and their supervisors than the issue of advocacy. Should we be advocates? Never? Sometimes? Always? And why is this such a controversial issue?

What does "advocacy" mean, anyway?

The dictionary tells us that an advocate is someone who speaks up on behalf of another. In healthcare interpreting, then, advocacy means stepping outside the role of facilitating understanding between two people speaking different languages in order to speak up on behalf of an individual (almost always a patient) who cannot assert his/her own important wishes or needs. Advocacy connotes conflict, or the potential for conflict. So, specifically, which of the following actions would constitute advocacy?

- Giving directions to the pharmacy?
  No, this is common courtesy.
- Offering your arm to an elderly patient who is going down some steps?
  Nope, that's courtesy again. There's no conflict, no need to speak up on someone's behalf.
- Informing a patient of his right to lodge a complaint?
  No, again, this is educating the patient about how the health care system in the U.S. works. It is not speaking up on his behalf, so it is not advocacy.

- Asking the receptionist to look again for an appointment next week, even though she says there are none, because the doctor specifically requested a 7-day follow-up?
  Yes, this is an act of advocacy. You are speaking up for the patient who is not speaking up for himself.
- Asking the provider if you can check to see if the patient understood because she looks confused to you?
  No, this is facilitating understanding in a communication; it is not advocacy.
- Intervening in an interpreted session because you perceive a cultural misunderstanding happening?
  Nope, you guessed it; this is facilitating understanding again.
- Seeking out the charge nurse in Labor and Delivery because you saw one of the OB nurses forge the patient's signature on a consent form for a C-section, a procedure that the patient has repeatedly refused?
  Yes, this is clearly an act of speaking up for someone who is unable to speak up for herself.

So, advocacy has nothing to do with helping a patient and provider understand each other, nor does it include acts of common courtesy or patient education. It does include speaking up for someone who cannot defend him or herself, in a situation in which a patient is not receiving adequate care.

When to advocate

Some knowledgeable people in this field insist that interpreters should never act as advocates, while others insist that at times they must. Both sides have reasonable arguments. Opponents of advocacy maintain that interpreters who speak up on behalf of the patient are no longer "neutral." They have taken sides and so are no longer objective and cannot be trusted by both parties to interpret accurately. Clearly, an interpreter who is advocating is no longer interpreting. Opponents also point out that advocating for patients can lead to patient dependency, can get the interpreter labeled as a troublemaker, can get the interpreter fired or blacklisted. Agencies may not pay for the time spent advocating, and the interpreter could even incur a degree of legal liability.

Supporters of interpreters as advocates counter by insisting that LEP patients often come from cultures and/or socioeconomic backgrounds in which problems are not resolved by "speaking up for oneself" and are therefore poorly equipped to manage problems in our health care system. They are likely to be unfamiliar with what to expect in our health care system and may not know their rights. Supporters also insist that many of the risks of advocating (dependency, getting labeled a troublemaker or blacklisted) can be managed if one advocates skillfully. It is simply a question of learning to advocate and mediate without causing division. And the final argument is the ethical one: as human beings, we cannot stand aside and see a patient put at risk, given poor care, or subjected to injustice without intervening.

So who is right?

The National Code of Ethics for Interpreters in Health Care states that "When the patient's health, well-being or dignity is at risk, an interpreter may be justified in acting as an advocate." The corresponding sections in the National Standards of Practice for Interpreters in Health Care are a bit more specific:

"31. The interpreter may speak out to protect an individual from serious harm.
32. The interpreter may advocate on behalf of a party or group to correct mistreatment or abuse."

Notice this is a careful statement that permits advocacy under certain conditions. This brings interpreting in line with other healthcare professions. After all, advocacy has its place in the role of **any** member of the healthcare team, whether it is the pediatrician, the head nurse, or the receptionist. However, it is a role we choose with care, keeping in mind the caveats mentioned above. Choosing whether or not to advocate in a particular situation depends on a series of factors, including:

- the policy of the agency you work for,
- the policy of the health care institution in which you are interpreting,
- how serious the outcome of not advocating would be,
- your knowledge of the particular health care setting in which you are interpreting,
- your relationship with the doctor/nurse/receptionist or whoever is the third person in the conflict.

(Oh, and by the way, because of the factors listed above, it is almost impossible to advocate effectively over the phone. So all you telephonic interpreters out there - feel free to take a break and get a cup of coffee.)

For you on-site interpreters, sooner or later you will be challenged by a situation in which you feel that the patient's health is being compromised, or in which you feel that the patient is not getting equal treatment or access. So here are some broad guidelines to help you decide whether or not to advocate and, if so, how to do so effectively and efficiently.

Do advocate if:

the patient is not getting the treatment to which he or she is entitled,

and

the potential consequences of the situation not being resolved are serious,

and

the patient wants you to advocate for him or her,

and

neither the agency you are working for nor the institution at which you are interpreting have specific prohibitions against advocating.

Do **not** advocate if:

the issue at hand is one of medical expertise, and it is clear that there has not been an oversight or misunderstanding,

or

the patient does not want to continue,

or

advocating would involve breaching confidentiality,

or

your agency or the institution for which you are interpreting has specifically prohibited interpreters from advocating.

How to advocate

As agency interpreters, you all probably have the most difficult starting point from which to advocate effectively. Since you are not employees of a given health care institution, and because you may interpret there only occasionally, it is hard to know exactly where to go to help a patient resolve a problem. For the same reasons, it is difficult to build the personal relationships with medical staff that can buy you some good will when mediating a conflict. Here are some suggestions then, adapted from the training program *Bridging the Gap*, on how to go about handling a situation in which you feel you need to speak up for someone who cannot speak up for herself.

1. Clearly identify the problem in your own mind.

2. Explain the problem to the patient, if you can. Ask the patient if he or she would like you to pursue the question.

3. Choose the person who is most likely to be able to address the problem. If possible, choose someone who already knows you.

4. Introduce yourself and the patient to the person whose help you need. Clearly and concisely explain the problem.

5. Ask questions to discover what options there are to solve the problem.

6. Avoid blaming, humiliating anyone, raising your voice, making threats, using sarcasm, contradicting anyone, interrupting. Take the attitude that you and the person you are addressing are teammates, working together to resolve the problem.

7. Use non-threatening language, such as "I am concerned about. . ." "I wonder if you could help me. . ."

8. Use non-threatening body language.

9. Bring your patient along on each step, if possible. Keep him or her in the loop as to what is happening.

Advocating is certainly not our primary role as interpreters. Some of us may rarely see situations that require advocacy. However, the potentially life-threatening nature of conflicts in the healthcare arena, coupled with the common and often enormous gulf between the power and preparation of healthcare providers/institutions and that of patients, means that interpreters in these venues must be ready to advocate if the patient's well-being is at stake. Far from making the interpreter unprofessional, knowing when and how to advocate is the hallmark of the interpreter as the newest professional member of the healthcare team.

August, 2003

11.

Sight Translation

What, When and How

Sight translation is the act of reading aloud in one language a text written in a different language. During any typical foray into the healthcare system, patients receive an abundance of documents to read, to fill out and/or to take home. While some hospitals invest in translating these documents for non-English speakers, most rely on the interpreter to read the document aloud to the patient, in the patient's language.

What sort of documents have you been called on to sight translate? How many can you think of?

Consent forms	Financial forms
Advance directives	HIPAA privacy rights
Admission forms	Patient history forms
Explanation of insurance	Discharge instructions
Medication instructions	Patient education materials
Preparation for surgery	Surveys
Dietary guides	Menus

Some of these documents, called "sender-oriented documents," are designed to meet the administrative or legal needs of the healthcare institution. Others, called "receiver-oriented documents," are designed to educate the patient so that he or she can participate in his or her own care.

In addition to the health facility's documents, an interpreter might be called upon to sight translate signage that could affect a patient's health care (e.g. signs in radiology asking patients to inform the technician if they could be pregnant), medicine packaging from the patient's country of origin, or medical documents from the patient's home country. In fact, patients in the U.S. healthcare system receive so much paperwork that at times it seems that an interpreter could spend hours sight translating it all. When, then, should a document be sight translated?

When should interpreters do sight translation?

In April 2009, the National Council on Interpreting in Health Care published a working paper dealing with an interpreter's role in doing either written or sight translation. You can download this document for free at www.ncihc.org. The guidelines in this working paper aim to strike a balance between the need to provide patients access to many written materials in many languages, and the difficulty in providing a really accurate sight translation of long or technical documents.

The NCIHC makes the following recommendations regarding when interpreters should take on a sight translation and when they should not.

- Documents that contain general background information (patient bill of rights, HIPAA forms) and educational materials are often quite long and so **are not appropriate** for sight translation. Sight translating these documents is both time consuming and probably fruitless, as the patient is unlikely to remember what was read to him.

- Documents with specific instructions **are appropriate** for sight translation, **with the provider present**, so that the patient's questions can be answered by the provider, not the interpreter.

- Legal documents, such as consent forms, **should be translated professionally** and then, if necessary, read aloud by the interpreter for the benefit of the client. There are several reasons for this recommendation. First, legal documents are usually written in complex and formal language, with many legal terms. Medical interpreters are often unfamiliar with this high register legal terminology and are at risk for rendering it inaccurately if required to translate it on site. In addition, it is questionable how much patients will understand and retain of what they simply hear in a long and complex sight translation. Finally, in accordance with The Joint Commission's standards for obtaining informed consent, providers are expected to explain the procedure to the patient, including risks and alternate options, and to ensure that the patient has understood the explanation. This means that, even with a translated consent form, a provider needs to be present while the patient reads the form (or the interpreter reads it to the patient), so as to answer questions and guide the interpreter if there is text that can be omitted (e.g. consent for anesthesia when none is going to be administered).[4]

How does an interpreter do sight translation?

Sight translation is not as easy as it looks. When sight translating, the interpreter cannot change the meaning of what is written, although it may be necessary to adapt sentence structure and vocabulary so that the message makes sense and sounds natural in the target language. Here are some steps for doing a quality sight translation.

1. Start by scanning the entire document. You are trying to understand the purpose and gist of the document, as well as looking for key vocabulary that you may not know. It is unfortunate that many healthcare documents are poorly written and confusing, making a sight translation even more difficult. Keep an eye out for multiple or vague meanings, for complex vocabulary and concepts, and for acronyms.

2. Ask for clarification of unfamiliar vocabulary or concepts before you start to sight translate.

3. Sight-translate a sentence at a time. Focus on translating idea by idea, not word for word, or you will get caught up in syntax. Be aware that you may have to change the order of the sentence so that it sounds natural in the target language; just make sure that you preserve the original meaning. Break long sentences into two shorter ones, so that they are easier to translate and easier to understand. Be careful of false cognates (words that sound alike between two languages but mean different things) and of inventing phrases that have no natural meaning in the target language.

4. Try to read at a normal and steady pace. As you're sight translating the first sentence, read ahead to the next sentence to ensure an even pace. It is difficult to listen to and understand a sight translation that has long gaps between sentences.

---

[4]*Sight Translation and Written Translation: Guidelines for Interpreters.* The National Council on Interpreting in Health Care, April 2009, pg. 7.

5. Sight-translate everything. Once you start to sight translate a document, you may not leave parts out, regardless of whether you feel them to be inappropriate or because you don't know the words. The only exception to this rule is when you translate forms. You may omit sections which are clearly not applicable to the particular patient's situation: for example, a section related to minors when the patient is an adult.

6. Refer questions to the provider. Patients may have questions about what they heard in the document. It is the provider's job to answer questions and explain concepts, not yours.

Other details:

After sight translating a document, you may be asked to sign, either as a witness or as the interpreter. It is entirely appropriate to sign a document as the interpreter, verifying that you sight translated the document for the patient. If you merely interpreted for the provider as he or she summarized the document, make sure you note that above the signature.

There is more ambivalence in the interpreter world about signing as a witness. Most professional interpreters decline to sign as witness, choosing instead to sign as the interpreter.

Sometimes, a sight translation is not enough. If you are asked to sight translate instructions (such as discharge instructions) to which a patient will need to refer later, it may be better to also provide a written translation. After all, no matter how good the sight translation was, who is going to remember three weeks later how to prepare for that colonoscopy? Do the written translation on the same page as the original English text so that they appear together; this way, if there is ever a question as to the accuracy of the translation, it will be easy to compare it to the original.

Sight translation is a complex skill that requires significant practice to master. Luckily, it is easy to practice just about anywhere. Whether it is the newspaper at the breakfast table or your children's bedtime storybooks, try sight translating the texts that fill your world. Soon you'll be able to help your limited-English-proficient patients make sense of the texts that fill theirs every time they come to the doctor.

April, 2006

Updated February, 2010

12.

Two Big Challenges:
Controlling Pacing and Handling Confrontation

Introduction

Interpreters encounter many challenges on a daily basis, from difficult content to difficult people. Two common ones are handling the flow of a session and handling the confrontation that can come up when an initially collaborative conversation becomes adversarial.

Handling the flow

In a perfect world, everyone who uses the services of an interpreter would speak in full thoughts and pause often so that you can interpret what has been said. Also in a perfect world, all interpreters would be skillful enough to remember long segments of speech and render the interpretation accurately and completely. Unfortunately, many people have never been taught to use an interpreter. As a result, you may find that some speakers speak without pause for quite a while, making it very difficult to do an accurate consecutive interpretation. In addition, many of us have not developed our memory skills enough, leading to a need for speakers to pause after every sentence, which is not reasonable. What to do? Here are a few suggestions:

1. **Start to interpret at pauses**
   You can help the speaker to know how long a segment of speech

you can handle by jumping in at a pause at the end of a thought. It is important to avoid the impression that you are interrupting, however. If the speaker does not fall into a comfortable rhythm fairly quickly, try the next technique.

2. **Ask the speaker to pause more often**
   Here's what it might sound like: "Speaking as the interpreter, I wonder if you could pause more often? That would really help me do a more accurate interpretation." Don't forget to let the other speaker on the line know what you just said.

3. **Take notes**
   One of the most useful skills you can learn as a telephone interpreter is note taking. Professional interpreters often develop their own sort of shorthand, based on symbols instead of words, that allows them to take notes quickly. The notes are not a transcription of what was said, but rather serve as a reminder, allowing you to accurately reproduce a much longer segment of speech than you could otherwise remember.

4. **Build memory skills.**
   If you often find yourself struggling to remember everything a speaker has said, you need to work on your memory skills. Simple exercises like having a friend read sentences to you and then repeating them back can help you stretch your short-term memory so that you can handle larger segments of speech without asking the speaker to pause.

As you know, accuracy and completeness are the cornerstones of good interpreting. Managing the flow allows you to interpret more completely, more accurately, and makes you a better interpreter.

Handling confrontation

Another challenge for telephone interpreters - and for all interpreters, really - is how to handle conversations in which one or more speakers become angry, upset, or even offensive. This probably happens most often on customer service calls (credit card collection calls, utilities, etc.) The key to handling this challenge is to remember that you are not the source of the message, only the means by which it is conveyed. Don't hold yourself responsible if people disagree, get angry, yell at each other, or even end the call on an unhappy, dissatisfied note. You are only responsible for making relatively sure that everything that was said was understood.

Still, it is hard to interpret for angry, upset people, especially when they may blame you for the way the call went. Here are a few suggestions:

1. Interpret everything, and be faithful to the content and tone of voice, but **underplay an angry or offensive tone.** That doesn't mean you should turn an angry response into a pleasant, polite response. It just means you should keep your tone of voice somewhat more moderate than the speaker.

2. **Remind all speakers that you will interpret everything** exactly as it was said. If a speaker challenges you about what you are interpreting, gently remind the speaker that you are interpreting faithfully everything that is being said.

3. **Stay calm and detached.** Staying detached means that you don't take personally anything that is said. After all, the two speakers are speaking (or yelling, as the case may be) at each other, not at you. Even if someone speaks sharply to you, the interpreter, remember that they are probably under a great deal of stress. Stay calm and polite in everything that you say for yourself, and don't let it bother you.

Over time, we hope that client education will reach everyone who uses interpreter services, so that speakers will not ramble on for minutes without pausing for interpretation, and so that speakers will not put interpreters in the middle of angry, confrontational discussions. Until that time, we need to hone our skills so that we can handle anything that comes our way in the calm, professional manner that befits a professional interpreter.

May, 2002

13.

Are You as Accurate as You Think You Are?

In July 2008 a truly worrisome article appeared in *Chest* Online, the official publication of the American College of Chest Physicians. This study,[5] conducted at a large, urban medical center, looked at medical interpreting in ICU family conferences regarding disconnecting life support or the sharing of bad news. Both the clinical interpreting and the subsequent translation of the recorded and transcribed encounters were done by Washington-State-certified medical interpreters. And for each interpreted exchange between clinicians and family, there was a 55% chance that an alteration would occur, 75% of which were judged by the researchers to be of potential clinical significance.

That means that, in any given exchange, the interpreters were more likely than not to make at least one serious error. And these guys were certified.

Why is this worrisome to me? While I do not know the individual interpreters involved in this study, I know the pool from which they were pulled. This particular hospital has, overall, one of the most well-trained and experienced groups of medical interpreters in the country. And yet, in this study they routinely made very serious

[5]Kiemanh Pham, J. Daryl Thornton, Ruth A. Engelberg, J. Carey Jackson and J. Randall Curtis. *Alterations During Medical Interpretations of ICU Family Conferences that Interfere or Enhance Communication.* Chest 2008; 134;109-116; Prepublished online March 17, 2008; DOI 10.1378/chest.07-2852, page 113-114.

errors. It is enough to make me go back and re-evaluate what I know about training interpreters. What does it say to you?

Consider what it means to be accurate as an interpreter. According to the National Code of Ethics for Interpreters in Health Care, accuracy means **"conveying the content and spirit of the original message, taking into consideration the cultural context."**[6] It means not adding, omitting or changing the meaning. While this sounds easy, this study suggests that interpreters - even certified interpreters - are not as successful at this as we had thought. So, let's look more closely at what it means to add, omit or change.

You are adding when you include any idea that the speaker did not say. This can be a sentence, a phrase, or a modifier. Interestingly, the researchers in this study found very few instances of simple additions in the interpretations. Of greater concern were omissions and changes of meaning.

You are omitting when you leave out any idea that the speaker did say. Here are some examples from the study:[7]

> Doctor: "I don't know what else to say to you. I mean, I told you yesterday that he's essentially brain dead. I don't know what you expected from that. I also said yesterday that there's no recovery from this."
>
> Interpreter: *"I told [you] that his brain was dead and it wasn't going to recover."*

> Here, the interpreter has significantly softened the harsh tone of the message by omitting some of the more brusque language. While the researchers considered this a positive change, from an interpreting point of view it is a change that the interpreter had no right to make.

> Doctor: "Does that sound like a good plan to you? Do you have any more questions?"
>
> Interpreter: "Do you agree?"

---

[6] *A National Code of Ethics for Interpreters in Health Care.* National Council on Interpreting in Health Care. July 2004, pg. 13.

[7] Kiemanh Pham, J. Daryl Thornton, Ruth A. Engelberg, J. Carey Jackson and J. Randall Curtis. *Alterations During Medical Interpretations of ICU Family Conferences that Interfere or Enhance Communication. Chest* 2008; 134;109-116; Prepublished online March 17, 2008; DOI 10.1378/chest.07-2852, page 113-114.

Here, the interpreter's alteration here has robbed the family of the chance to express doubt and ask questions, as well as perhaps impacting the rapport between family and provider.

You are substituting when you include an idea that is different from what the speaker says.

From the study: [8]

Doctor: "I don't know. Um, this is a very rapidly progressing cancer."

Interpreter: *"He doesn't know because it starts gradually."*

Here the interpretation is the exact opposite of the original message, leaving the family with a serious misconception about the patient's illness that may affect the decisions they make on the patient's behalf.

Doctor: "Have you spoken to your husband about these kinds of questions before he got sick, what his wishes might be in this sort of situation?"

Interpreter: *"Did you talk to your husband before he got so sick about possible situations, what was awaiting him?"*

The provider was trying to get a sense of the patient's wishes for his end-of-life care. The interpreter has changed the wording so the emphasis was on the patient's perception of his illness. This may make it harder for the provider and family to agree on a treatment plan that actually reflects the patient's wishes.

Family: *"But, what we want to know is that after his lungs get better and when he wakes up will his brain suffer and affect his ability to recognize people?"*

Interpreter: "Okay, she wants to know about the lungs, when he wakes up, so about his lungs, and so, what about after, so it will not affect him?"

---

[8] ibid

Here, the provider understood the family to be asking about the prognosis of the patient's respiratory function. He never realized that the family was asking about the patient's likely neurological status.

Doctor: "The problem with this option is that he may have to stay on this machine for the rest of his life."

Interpreter: *"But the problem with this option is that he will have to stay on this machine for the rest of his life."*

This simple change from "may" to "will" could have a significant impact on the family's decision as to whether to place this patient on a respirator.

Of course, it is easy to look at a written transcript and see errors, and not so easy to be accurate during the stress of an oral interpretation. But the alterations cited above are extremely serious; one can easily see how they might change the course of a family's decisions for a dying loved one. If interpreters want to be viewed as professionals, this level of performance is not acceptable.

So, how about you? Maybe you think that you are already very accurate in your interpreting. Or maybe you feel that most of your interpreting is in venues where a few mistakes won't make any difference. Or maybe you feel that since you don't interpret full time, you're not a "real" interpreter and these concerns don't apply to you.

If you're thinking that a few mistakes don't matter, think again. Sloppy interpreting becomes a habit and is never acceptable. And if you think that you're already pretty accurate, here's a challenge for you: write up a dialogue based on your interpreting experiences, sit down with a friend to read the patient's and provider's parts, and tape record it. Then listen to your own interpreting and check your accuracy. Seriously consider the consequences of the changes you introduce into the messages. And then find ways to practice. Notice that none of the errors in the study stemmed from not knowing medical terminology; they were errors in conversion alone.

Healthcare interpreting is moving from being an ad-hoc activity to a real profession. National certification is just around the corner. This is no longer an activity for people who simply want something to do between jobs, but a serious endeavor that has critical implications for medical care. We can't afford to be omitting or changing the message when we interpret. This study in *Chest* is a wake-up call to all of us who interpret or train interpreters. I'm certainly going to reconsider what I emphasize in my training programs. How about you? Will you reconsider how you do *your* work? Twenty-six million LEP patients and all the health providers in the country are depending on us to do just that.

August 2008

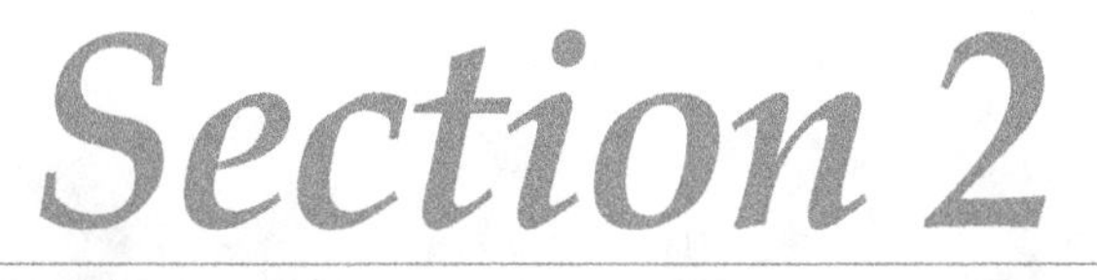

The Key to Success: Being Prepared!

14.

Not Child's Play

Interpreting in Pediatrics

The whole family's there, and everybody's talking at once. Some speak English and some do not. The baby is crying. You trip over the toys that got dropped on the floor. The patient is four years old and adorable and dying.

Never has interpreting seemed less like a walk in the park.

Interpreting in pediatrics has all of the challenges of interpreting for adults and then some. And while we do not yet have specialized training and certification for interpreting for children, it would make sense. After all, doctors have to specialize to treat children; teachers get a special certificate to teach children. So, when interpreting for children, there are some particular issues to keep in mind.

Establishing rapport with children

You're sick, you're in a strange place, you're surrounded by people you don't know, and Mom and Dad look upset and worried. How much scarier can it get?

As interpreters, we know that pre-sessions are always important in helping to establish rapport with patients. When interpreting in pediatrics, it is important to introduce yourself to the parents of the patient first, and then to the child as well. Younger children may not respond to your introduction, but a warm smile and greeting is reassuring and will help them trust you. Don't attempt to touch a child unless there is a specific reason to do so.

If the child is old enough that the provider may be asking him or her questions directly, it is also important to explain your role to the child in terms he or she can understand. Of course, how you do this will depend on the patient's age. Older children may "get" that you are repeating the doctor's words, or Mom's words, or their words in the other language. Younger children, however, may be more likely to talk directly to you, instead of to the provider. In this case, you may have to switch from first person to reported speech when addressing the child in order to facilitate clear communication. In the same way, you may need to position yourself where the child can see you, and make eye contact when you interpret to the child.

Controlling the flow

Controlling the flow of the conversation is a greater challenge in pediatrics for two reasons. First of all, there tend to be more people present in these interactions. Except with adolescent children, there is always at least one parent present, and sometimes there are many family members in the room. Some may speak English, while others don't. Here are some guidelines for handling these situations.

- Ask the provider at the beginning of the session to request that only one person speak at a time, so that you can interpret accurately.

- If everyone is talking at once, just stop interpreting and wait for them all to be quiet.

- If one person after another speaks, use your open hand to gesture at the person for whom you are interpreting at any given moment.

- If the patient is speaking English to the doctor, switch to simultaneous mode to interpret the speech for the parents. If the parents then wish to respond, switch back to consecutive mode.

- If the doctor asks a question of the child and the parent answers, interpret the parent's speech and let the doctor clarify if he or she wants the child to answer.

The second reason that flow becomes an issue is that kids often forget that they're supposed to pause for the interpreter. This is not a big problem, as most children respond in short segments anyway. In the unlikely event that you get a young patient who is truly loquacious, your best bet is to take good notes from which to interpret when the child stops speaking.

Child speech

A child's control of speech is still developing into adolescence. For this reason, pediatricians choose their words carefully when talking to a child, in order to pitch the register at a level that the child can understand. You must do the same. In addition, your rendering of the child's speech should reflect the level of speech the child is using. That will help the doctor assess the child's development and know how to pitch his or her own responses.

Self-care

The final challenge of interpreting for children is dealing with your own feelings. It is normal to feel particularly protective of children; that is why we find a child's illness or death so heart-wrenching. In pediatrics - especially in the sub-specialties - you may see kids who are experiencing a lot of pain and suffering. You may wish you could hug them, or do something special to help them. How do you handle that?

Maintaining a professional boundary is especially important in pediatrics. Your role with the child is not that of parent or caregiver: it is to facilitate communication. While interpreters can and should be warm and friendly, take care not to get overly involved with a particular child or family. And make sure you have some mechanism outside of work to deal with your own sadness about the suffering of the children for whom you interpret. Some interpreters find release in physical activity, some in prayer, others in artistic outlets. Keep in mind that your presence in itself is an incredible support to these children and families, because you give them access to health care as nobody else could.

Of course, sometimes your feelings for the children for whom you interpret may not be so tender. Maintaining a professional demeanor when some cute little tot kicks you in the shin is just as important. And that long run when you get home works just as well.

Interpreting in pediatrics is certainly not child's play. However, if you keep in mind your basic purpose - to facilitate understanding in communication - you will find the best way to adjust your technique to whatever situation presents itself.

January, 2005

15.

Interpreting in the Asthma Clinic

About 20 million people in the U.S. have been diagnosed with it.

9 million of these are children.[9]

In 2003, 4099 people died of it.

The following year, the condition led to 1.8 million Emergency Room visits.

That same year, it cost the U.S. $16.1 billion in healthcare expenditures and lost productivity.[10]

If you haven't interpreted for a case yet, you will soon.

Asthma. When I was growing up, people saw it as a sign of "weak lungs" or just a case of really bad seasonal allergies. But now, even the general public is coming to understand that asthma is a potentially serious condition affecting a growing number of people. In some communities it has become all too common; for example, five percent

[9] National Heart Lung and Blood Institute

[10] American Lung Association

of Hispanic children are reported to suffer from the condition.[11] While asthma has no cure, it can be effectively controlled. This depends on a great deal of patient education, which in turn depends on clear communication between providers, patients, and, when the patient is a child, the patient's family. When either the patient or the family is limited English proficient, effective interpreting becomes critical in the process of teaching the patient how to recognize and manage symptoms. As interpreters then, we must understand asthma, so that we can interpret accurately.

What is asthma?

Asthma is an inflammation of the inner lining of the airways in the lungs, which causes them to be very sensitive to anything that can cause irritation. When the airways react to those irritants, the lining swells, narrowing the airway and making it hard to breathe. Sometimes the muscles surrounding the bronchial passages also tighten and an especially thick mucus is excreted inside the air passages. When all these symptoms get suddenly worse and impede normal breathing, it is called an asthma attack. If the inflammation and the tightening muscles and mucus combine to shut off the flow of air altogether, the patient can die.

What causes an asthma attack? The triggers differ for different people and may include:

- Allergens, such as pollen, dust, animal dander, mold, etc.
- Air-borne irritants, such as dust, cigarette smoke, air pollution, strong odors, sudden changes in air temperature
- Some medications, such as aspirin and beta-blockers
- Some food additives, such as the sulfites which are found in dried fruit and wine
- Some diseases, such as respiratory infections or gastroesophageal reflux disease
- Stress
- Extreme bouts of crying or laughing
- Exercise

During an asthma attack, the patient can experience a variety of symptoms:

- Difficulty breathing, especially a sense that he can't get enough air in and out of his lungs
- Chest pain or pressure
- Wheezing (a whistling or squeaky sound when he breathes)
- Coughing, more at night and in the early morning
- Very noisy breathing

[11] U.S. Environmental Protection Agency

When a patient presents with a history of these sorts of symptoms, physicians may do any of a number of tests to confirm a diagnosis. One of these is a pulmonary function test, which measures how well the lungs are working. The patient will be asked to breathe in as deeply as possible and then to blow out as long as he can into a tube attached to a machine. This machine will measure the volume of air the lungs can handle and the speed at which the lungs can exhale it (called "peak flow"). The physician may also request a chest X-ray, to check for other pulmonary conditions, and skin tests to identify possible triggers such as allergies.

Managing Asthma

As mentioned earlier, there is no cure for asthma, although some children seem to grow out of it. Since asthma can reappear at any time, treatment focuses on both responding to attacks when they occur and managing the condition long term. Let's look first at that frightening experience called an asthma attack.

An asthma attack is an acute event that requires immediate attention. Patients with asthma often carry a bronchodilator, usually in the form of an inhaler, that can relax the muscles that are constricting the bronchial tubes, allowing more air to pass and relieving the awful inability to breathe. In severe attacks, however, the bronchodilator may not be sufficient, and the patient may need to seek immediate medical attention.

Over the long term, patients and their families can take a number of measures to lower the frequency and severity of asthma symptoms.

1. **Triggers** need to be reduced or removed from the environment, especially at home.

   For example, washing pets weekly minimizes pet dander, removing items like carpeting or stuffed animals can cut down on dust, and installing air conditioning can help maintain a clean-air environment. Some patients, for whom the trigger was a chemical common to their workplace, have had to change jobs to control their asthma.

2. **Medications** can relieve symptoms during an attack or decrease the frequency of attacks.

   Medications are divided into two groups based on their function. The first group includes the long-term daily controllers. These are anti-inflammatories, used daily to control inflammation in the airways and making them less sensitive to triggers. This prevents asthma flare-ups. The most common of these medicines are corticosteroids such as Advair, Flovent, QVAR and Pulmicort, and the non-steroidal

Singulair.

The other group contains the quick-relief or "rescue" medicines. They are also called bronchodilators or beta-agonists. They ease breathing during an asthma attack by relaxing the muscles that are clamping down on the airways. The more common of these are albuterol (ProAir, Proventil, Ventolin), Xopenex and Maxair.

3. **Peak flow monitoring**
   Patients can track how well they are breathing by monitoring peak flow on a daily basis at home with a peak flow meter. The peak flow meter is a hand-held, portable device that measures how open the airways are. The patient takes a big breath in, puts the mouthpiece in his mouth and then blows out as fast and as hard as possible. The patient can then read on the meter how much air he was able to exhale. If peak flow starts to decrease, this is a sign that his airways are constricting and that an attack may be coming on. In response, the patient can use a bronchodilator and avert the attack before it becomes a crisis. Removing any triggers will help ease asthma symptoms and avoid an imminent attack.

4. **Exercise**
   While extreme exercise can trigger asthma attacks in many people, moderate exercise to improve the overall health of heart, lungs and body can often help in the long run.

Controlling asthma is especially important during pregnancy. During asthma attacks, less oxygen reaches the blood, and that means less oxygen is reaching the developing baby too. Most asthma medicines are safe to take during pregnancy.

Older patients must also take care in controlling their asthma. The higher doses of steroids used to control bronchial inflammation long term can also lower bone density, so older patients on corticosteroids may need to also take vitamin D and calcium. In addition, some medications such as beta-blockers and aspirin that are commonly used to treat high blood pressure, and non-steroidal anti-inflammatory drugs used to treat arthritis, can interfere with asthma medications or even cause asthma attacks.

Further Study

To learn more about asthma, check out the following sites. Then see if you can define and translate the vocabulary that follows.

- Medline Plus at http://medlineplus.gov/
- The American Lung Association at: http://www.lungusa.org/site/pp.asp?c=dvLUK9O0E&b=33316
- The National Heart Lung and Blood Institutes of the National Institutes for Health, part of the U.S. Department of Health and Human Services, at http://www.nhlbi.nih.gov/health/dci/Diseases/Asthma

acute (adjective)
additives (food additives)
airways
allergen
alveolus (plural = alveoli)
asthma
attack
bronchi
bronchioles
bronchodilator
carbon dioxide
chronic (adjective)
cilia
constrict (verb)
dander (animal dander)
dust mites
inflammation
inhaler
irritants (air-borne irritants)
larynx
lining
metered-dose inhaler
mucus
narrow (verb)
nebulizer
peak flow
peak flow meter
puff
pulmonary function test
relax (verb)
rescue inhaler
secrete (verb)
skin test for allergies
spacer
stress
swell (verb)
trachea
trigger (verb)
trigger (noun)
wheezing

Conclusion

Asthma can be pretty scary for those who suffer from it. But with clear interpreting, limited-English-proficient patients can learn to manage their asthma so that it does not unduly impact their lives.

February 2010

16.

A Prescription for Accuracy

Interpreting in the Pharmacy

Language Access in commercial pharmacies

I have always wondered when it would happen. Much attention has been paid over the past two decades to providing language access in hospitals and clinics, but I wondered when someone would notice that commercial pharmacies, which also accept federal funding in the form of Medicaid and Medicare, do not as a rule provide interpreters for patients who do not speak English. Isn't it a concern that millions of LEP patients are getting their medications without knowing how to take them correctly? Apparently it is, at least in New York.

Over the past two years, the Attorney General of New York has been investigating complaints against six national chain pharmacies, which complainants say "routinely fail to advise non-English speaking customers in a language that allows them to understand the purpose, dosage, and side-effects of their medications."[12] As of this writing, all six companies have entered into agreements with the AG's office which should lead to significant increases in language assistance, not only at the chains'

[12] Press release from the Office of the Attorney General of New York State: *Cuomo announces agreements with two of the nation's largest pharmacies to provide customers with prescription medication instructions in their primary language.* November 13, 2008

pharmacies in New York, but in their pharmacies across the country.

And last week, the New York City Council voted the agreements into civil law, applicable to all pharmacies in the city.

Neither the AG's office nor the New York City Council are dictating how the pharmacies must provide language assistance, but most will be making use of telephonic interpreting services. So telephonic interpreters across the country will likely be seeing an increase in the number of pharmacy calls they receive. These calls are likely to be relatively short (5-7 minutes) and relatively straightforward. However short and straightforward, though, this is high-stakes interpreting for sure, because an error can be more than serious; it can be deadly.

A typical medication counseling session

If you interpret for a commercial pharmacy, you will most likely be interpreting the counseling that a pharmacist does with patients when they pick up a medication that is new for them. The pharmacist will probably address the following topics:

1. **Name and class of medication**

   Interpret classes of medication (e.g. antidepressants=*antidepresivos* in Spanish), but not the name of the medication (Zoloft). Exceptions are the very common medications whose converted names have become commonly recognized in the non-English language (e.g. penicillin=*penicilina*, aspirin=*aspirina*).

   Why does it seem that some medications have two names? For example, you can purchase Motrin and Ibuprofen, and the ingredients on the box look the same. In fact, they are, and this is a good example of what happens with virtually all pharmaceuticals today. When ibuprofen (the **chemical name**) was first developed, the pharmaceutical company patented that compound under the **brand name** Motrin. For the duration of the patent, no other company could produce that medication, and patients could only purchase Motrin. When the patent expired, other companies began to produce ibuprofen, marketing it under its chemical name; these are called **generic drugs.** So now you can purchase Motrin or ibuprofen. Chemically, they are exactly the same, but the generic drug is routinely cheaper.

2. Indications

Indications are what the medication is generally used for. For example, prednisone (name) is a corticosteroid (class) used, among other things, to reduce inflammation caused by rheumatoid arthritis (indication).

3. Action

What does the medication do in the body? How does it work? For example, Atenolol (name) is a beta-blocker (class) used to treat high blood pressure (indication) because it decreases the activity of the heart by blocking the beta receptors in the cardiac muscle (action).

4. Dosage, timing and mode of administration

How much of the medication should the patient take? When should he take it, and how? This is the most important information for the patient to remember, and accuracy in this part of the interpretation is absolutely critical. Here are some of the most common instructions around mode of administration.

"Take the capsule (or tablet or pill) . . . . "
Pay special attention if the pharmacist indicates that the tablets are to be taken sub-lingually (that is, not swallowed but placed under the tongue) or bucally (not swallowed, but allowed to dissolve in the mouth). Some tablets need to be broken in half, some need to be chewed, some can be crushed and mixed with a liquid.

"Insert the suppository. "
Suppositories are inserted into the anus after removing the wrapping.

"Take two puffs from the inhaler."
Inhalers can be designed to be used orally (through the mouth) or nasally (through the nose).

"Put two dropper-fulls in the baby's ear."

"Apply the ointment (or cream)."

"Give the injection."
Injections are given either subcutaneously (under the skin), intradermally (in the skin), intramuscularly (in the muscle), or intravenously (in the vein). There's a big difference among the four, so if the pharmacist specifies the mode of injection, make sure the patient understands it.

"Take the elixir (solution, suspension, syrup)."
Pharmaceutically speaking, these are four different modes of delivering a medication, however, from the patient's point of view, they are all just swallowed.

"Put on the patch."
A transdermal drug delivery system (TDDS), more commonly referred to as a patch, delivers medication slowly over time through the skin.

"Give the enema."

"Insert the vaginal cream using the applicator."

5. **Effect**

Pharmacists will also tell the patient what to expect after taking the medication. How long will it be until the medicine takes effect? What will the patient experience as the medication does its work?

6. **Possible drug interactions**

Pharmacists may ask about what other medications a patient is taking, in order to assure that there are no potential drug interactions with the prescribed medication. Please note that when the pharmacist asks for other medications, she is really interested in anything the patient might be taking that is pharmaceutically active. So, in addition to other prescribed meds, she also wants to know about any herbal medications, naturopathic mixtures, and dietary supplements that the patient may be taking.

7. **Possible side effects and adverse reactions**

Side effects are those secondary effects of the medication that are to be expected. An anticoagulant will make a cut bleed longer, many contraceptive pills will lead to weight gain. Adverse reactions are secondary effects of a medication that are not expected, that are rare and often serious; some anti-depressants can lead to worsening of depression, but not often; diuretics can lead to severe dehydration, but that is unusual.

Altogether, counseling from a pharmacist to a patient might sound like this:

"This medication is called hydrochlorothiazide, or HCTZ for short. It's a diuretic, commonly used to treat high blood pressure by increasing the amount of urine you make and so decreasing the amount of fluid you've got in your body. Less fluid means lower pressure, kind of like having less water in a hose. You're only taking 25 mg., which is a fairly low dosage. You need to take one tablet once a day. It's best to take this in the morning, since it's going to make you pee more than usual. If you take it at dinnertime or bedtime, you're likely to be up several times at night going to the bathroom.

"One thing to be careful of is that this medicine will make you particularly sensitive to direct sunlight, so if you go out in the sun, be sure to cover up or use a high SPF sunscreen.

"Are you taking any other medications, supplements, or herbal remedies? Generally, this medication is tolerated well, but call your doctor right away if you suddenly start getting muscle cramps or weakness, dizziness, an irregular heartbeat or an unusual decrease in the amount of urine you produce.

"So, one a day, in the morning, expect to urinate more than usual, and stay out of the sun. Any questions?"

Further study

If you would like to improve your ability to interpret in the pharmacy, or if you just find pharmaceuticals interesting, a great resource is the *Guide to Common Medications, Second Edition 2008*, available from the Cross Cultural Health Care Program at http://www.xculture.org.

Many thanks to David Schiesser, B.S.Pharm, Pharmacy Manager, Richmond Beach Quality Food Centers, for his input for this article.

September 2009

17.

The Language of Consent

Sight Translating the Hospital Consent Form

The use of consent forms in medicine in the U.S. grew out of two interesting movements in the dominant culture, both of which grew more prevalent during the 1970's. The first was a shift in the role of the physician from the "all-knowing deity" who told a patient what to do, to an expert advisor who provided information to patients about their options. The new paradigm saw patients as "health care consumers" or "part of the health care team" who ought to make their own decisions about what health care they wanted. The second movement was a legal one that saw more and more doctors being sued for malpractice when health outcomes were not what patients had hoped for or expected.

Consequently, consent forms in the U.S. health care system have come to fulfill two functions. When applied correctly, they assure that the patient has sufficient information to make a real choice as to whether he or she wants a particular procedure done. The form aims to insure that the patient understands the procedure, the risks entailed and the alternatives available, so that the patient can make an informed decision. The other purpose, of course, is to protect the doctor and the health care institution should legal action be taken as the result of an unexpected negative outcome.

Paradoxically, then, the consent form aims to be both an educational document and a legal document. Sometimes it seems that these two purposes are at odds with each other. From an interpreter's point of view, it makes it hard to know whether this is a collaborative (educational) interaction, allowing more explanation, or whether this is an adversarial (legal) interaction, requiring strict adherence to the conduit role. Unfortunately, given the ambiguity, we must deal with consent forms as legal documents, interpreting strictly and only what is on the page or what is stated by the provider during an oral consent.

What makes consent forms difficult is partially the terminology, but more so the register. Consent forms are most often written in the passive voice, with complicated sentence structure and long strings of dependent clauses. It is crucial, then, to read a paragraph through before you interpret it. If the target language does not have the passive voice construction, you will have to identify a subject (stated or implied). You may have to break long, convoluted sentences into shorter sentences. You must be very careful to conserve the same meaning. Where possible, maintain the same register.

In the first column of the following box, you'll find the complete text of a sample consent form. This one is written in a higher register than others I've seen. In the second column, I've included a lower register explanation of what this paragraph means. After reading the two columns, practice sight translating the original consent, using the points mentioned in the previous paragraph. If you can handle this form, you'll be fine with others of lower register.

One final comment about consent forms. If you are interpreting in person and you are handed a consent form to sight translate, you **must** translate everything on the page. You may be asked to sign the form, verifying that you interpreted it. In this case, you should sign **only** if you have translated the entire document.[13] If you have interpreted an oral consent by the physician (that is, if the physician summarizes the form orally instead of having you read the whole thing), you should add a note specifically stating that you have interpreted an oral consent administered by Dr. Whoever-it-is. If there is ever a legal question about whether the patient understood the procedure, you want to make sure that it is clear whether you sight translated the whole document, or, at the physician's direction, interpreted only a summary of what was in the document.

[13] If you are asked to sign as a witness, cross out the word "witness" and write in "interpreter."

Text of a Sample Consent Form

By my signature, I hereby authorize Dr. __________________ and/or such associates or assistants as may be selected by said physician, to treat the following condition(s) which has (have) been explained to me: (the doctor should have written in here the patient's diagnosis).

The procedures planned for treatment of my condition(s) have been explained to me by my physician. I understand them to be: (*the doctor should have written in here the specific treatment or procedure to which the patient is being asked to agree*).

I recognize that, during the course of the operation, post-operative care, medical treatment, anesthesia or other procedure, unforeseen conditions may necessitate additional or different procedures than those above set forth. I therefore authorize my above named physician, and his or her assistants or designees, to perform such surgical or other procedures as are in the exercise of his, her or their professional judgment necessary and desirable. The authority granted under this paragraph shall extend to the treatment of all conditions that require treatment and are not known to my physician at the time the medical or surgical procedure is commenced.

I have been informed that there are significant risks such as severe loss of blood, infection and cardiac arrest that can lead to death or permanent or partial disability, which may be attendant to the performance of any procedure.

Continued, next page

Lower Register

By signing this document, I am giving my permission for Dr. __________________ to treat me for the medical problem that is described here. I am also giving my permission for this treatment to be done by anyone that this doctor chooses to help or replace him. The doctor has explained my medical problem to me.

My doctor has explained to me the treatment for my medical problem. I understand that she will treat me by doing what is written here:

I understand that something may happen during the operation, during my care after the operation, during medical treatment, or during the use of anesthesia, that will make it necessary for the doctor to do some other procedure that isn't listed here. I give my permission to my doctor to do any other procedure that he believes is necessary. I also give my permission for the other people that are helping or replacing my doctor to do any other procedures that they think are necessary. This permission covers anything that comes up during the procedure, even if my doctor didn't know about it when he started.

My doctor has explained that there are serious risks involved in any procedure. They might include losing a lot of blood, getting an infection, or having a heart attack. These problems could lead to death, or to becoming partly or permanently disabled. I recognize that nobody has promised me that the

Continued, next page

I acknowledge that no warranty or guarantee has been made to me as to result or cure.

I consent to the administration of anesthesia by my attending physician, by an anesthesiologist, or other qualified party under the direction of a physician as may be deemed necessary. I understand that all anesthetics involve risks of complications and serious possible damage to vital organs such as the brain, heart, lung, liver and kidney and that in some cases may result in paralysis, cardiac arrest, and/or brain death from both known and unknown causes.

I consent to the transfusion of blood and blood products as deemed necessary.

Any tissues or parts surgically removed may be disposed of by the hospital or physician in accordance with accustomed practice.

I certify that my physician has informed me of the nature and character of the proposed treatment, of the anticipated results of the proposed treatment, of the possible alternative forms of treatment, and the recognized serious possible risks, complications, and the anticipated benefits involved in the proposed treatment and the alternative forms of treatment, including non-treatment.

I certify this form has been fully explained to me, that I have read it or had it read to me, that the blank spaces have been filled in, and that I understand its contents.

treatment will be successful or that I will be cured.

I give my permission for my doctor, an anesthesiologist, or any other qualified person working under my doctor's supervision, to give me anesthesia. I understand that there are risks involved in having anesthesia. I understand that the anesthesia could result in damage to my brain, heart, lungs, liver and kidney. I understand that it could even cause paralysis, heart attack or brain death, due to reasons that the doctors may not understand.

I give my permission for the doctors to give me a blood transfusion or other blood products (like plasma) if they think it is necessary.

I give permission for the doctors or hospital to do whatever they normally do with anything they remove from my body during the procedure.

I agree that my doctor has told me about the treatment that I'm going to have. He's told me about the results that he expects from the treatment and about other possible treatments. He's told me about the possible complications, the possible risks, and the possible benefits from this treatment and from other possible forms of treatment, including no treatment at all.

I agree that my doctor has explained to me everything on this form. I have read the form, or it has been read to me. All the blanks on the form have been filled in. I understand what is written here.

18.

The ABCs of DNA

Interpreting for Genetic Counseling

There are many ways in which interpreting assignments can be difficult. Sometimes the news you are conveying is bad; sometimes the people you are interpreting for are frustrating; sometimes the linguistic conversion is a challenge. And sometimes the material you are interpreting is so technically complex that just understanding what the provider said is tricky.

This last is often the case with genetic counseling appointments. Genetics is a relatively new science that even many well-educated people find difficult to understand. However, as scientists come to understand more of how genetics impacts health, more patients receive genetic counseling. Genetic screening has become common, for example, for pregnant women whose fetuses are at risk for birth defects. Conveying the concepts discussed in these counseling sessions can be challenging. For that reason, instead of the usual list of vocabulary words to learn and translate, this article will go into a bit more depth on genetic issues. The better we as interpreters understand these concepts, the more accurately we can interpret them.

DNA, Genes and Chromosomes

At the very heart of every cell of any living creature is a genetic code that determines what that cell will do and become, and what role it will play in the overall organism of which that cell is a part. The genetic code is built into the DNA (deoxyribonucleic acid), which takes the form of a double helix. If you've never seen a picture of DNA, imagine a tiny ladder made of flexible rubber; hold each end of the ladder in one hand and twist one end around and around. The resulting spiral ladder looks like DNA. A strand of DNA makes up a gene, and packets of genes are called chromosomes.

Generally, human beings have 23 pairs of chromosomes, each of which carries the genes that determine the individual traits of the person to which they belong. However, unlike all the other cells in a human body, an egg and a sperm carry only one chromosome of each pair. The egg and sperm join during fertilization, restoring the total of 46 chromosomes, and creating a unique genetic code. The fertilized egg then reproduces itself, over and over, growing eventually into an embryo, a fetus, and then a totally distinctive individual.

How Genetic Abnormalities Happen

Several things can go wrong with this process. Sometimes an altered gene that causes illness is passed from the mother or father to the child. In these *single gene disorders,* the number of chromosomes is normal, but some mutated gene within one of the chromosomes causes the genetic disorder in the child. Cystic fibrosis is an example of a single gene disorder.

Chromosomal disorders are problems stemming from an abnormal number or arrangement of chromosomes. For example, the genes within the chromosomes are normal, but instead of 46 normal chromosomes, there may be more or less. Down syndrome (or trisomy 21) is an example of a chromosomal disorder. How does this happen?

Most cells in the human body have 46 chromosomes (23 pairs). The egg and the sperm, however, are special cells that have only 23 chromosomes: one of each pair. They are formed during a complex cell division process called *meiosis.*

Sometimes during meiosis, a mistake happens. As the original germ cell divides in the process of becoming a sperm (for example), both of the chromosomes in a pair may end up in only one of the resulting sperm; the other receives none of that chromosome at all. When any one of these abnormal sperm joins with a normal egg, the fertilized egg ends up with either three of a particular chromosome (*trisomy*) or only one (*monosomy*).

Trisomy and monosomy are not normal conditions and most often lead to miscarriage or, if the fetus lives to term, to anatomical or developmental abnormalities. Even just a fragment of an extra chromosome (*a marker chromosome*) or a pattern of extra chromosomes in some cells but not others (*mosaicism*) may lead to a disorder in the child. On the other hand, genetic testing is a young science, and there is much we still do not understand about how genetic code is expressed in human development. While marker chromosomes and mosaicism cause abnormal conditions in some individuals, in others they seem to have no visible impact at all.

Doctors have found that genetically normal women who first become pregnant later in life are at greater risk of having a child with a chromosomal abnormality. For this reason, doctors routinely send first-time mothers over the age of 35 for routine genetic screening. They will also refer women with a history of genetically related health problems, women who already have one child with a genetic disorder, and women who have had two or more miscarriages. This allows the parents to find out if the fetus is affected and if so, to decide whether to terminate the pregnancy. If the parents choose to carry the pregnancy to term, this early knowledge helps them prepare the special care the child will need after he or she is born.

Genetic Screening

There are a number of tests that can be done as part of genetic screening.

1. **Maternal serum screening tests** are blood tests that check the levels of various substances associated with genetic defects. The triple screen measures alpha-fetoprotein (AFP), beta human chorionic gonadotropin (beta-hCG), and a type of estrogen (unconjugated estriol, or uE3). The quad screen checks these substances and the level of the hormone inhibin A. Alpha-fetoproteins are the first proteins that form the basis of blood in an embryo; when found to be elevated in amniotic fluid, they can be a sign of fetal anencephaly (lack of a brain) or open neural tube defects like spina bifida. The triple screen is usually done through a blood test at around 16-18 weeks but can also be done during the first trimester together with an ultrasound to identify potential problems.

2. **Ultrasound** can be used very early on in pregnancy to screen for certain traits such as nuchal thickening that are associated with certain genetic defects.

3. **Chorionic Villus Sampling** is a method for diagnosis of fetal diseases by sampling the cells of the placenta for DNA analysis. This test can be carried out as early as the 10th week of pregnancy. However, abnormal results are not definitive, as trisomy or monosomy may be due to errors in the chromosomal separation that happened after the cells that became the placenta had already differentiated from those forming the fetus. Therefore a positive CVS result will need to be

followed by an amniocentesis.

4. **Amniocentesis** is a method for diagnosis of fetal diseases by sampling the fluid in the amniotic sac for DNA analysis. This test is usually carried out between the 12th and 14th weeks of pregnancy. This test is more definitive, as the amniotic fluid contains cells that have sloughed off the skin of the actual fetus.

The greatest difficulty with genetic screening is that the science of detection has outpaced the association of meaning. So geneticists may identify an "abnormality" and still not know what it means for the child who carries it. Certain abnormalities, however, are well documented.

Impact of Genetic Abnormalities

As a rule, most fetuses that have genetic abnormalities are miscarried; genetic defects are found in over 50% of miscarriages. While trisomy can occur in any chromosome, only trisomy 21 (Down syndrome), trisomy 13 (Patau syndrome), trisomy 18 (Edward syndrome), and trisomies of the sex chromosomes have been documented in live births. Fetuses with monosomy are virtually always miscarried, excepting only a very few with monosomy X (Turner syndrome).

Interpreting for Genetic Counseling

Interpreting for genetic counseling is difficult on many fronts. If you don't understand what the provider is saying, intervene to ask for clarification. If the overall register is too high and if you sense that the patient is lost, tell the provider you'd like to ask the patient what she understood of what was just said. This method is called "teach back" and is a recognized technique in medical interviewing. If the provider is getting frustrated because you are taking a long time to build word pictures of these concepts, let the provider know that there are no linguistic – or even conceptual -- equivalents for these words in the patient's language.

Finally, if you interpret often for genetic counseling, study on your own about this topic. One useful resource is Genetics Home Reference (http://ghr.nlm.nih.gov/) from the National Institutes of Health. To help in learning the vocabulary of genetics, check out the *Talking Glossary of Genetic Terms*, NIH (National Human Genome Research Institute) which is also available in Spanish. The more you learn, the easier it will be to make the alphabet soup of genetic counseling into a palatable experience for the patient, the counselor, and for yourself.

June 2007

19.

Behavioral Health Interpreting – Part I

Behavioral health, sometimes called mental health, is quite an extensive field, including services that are provided to a broad range of patients in a broad range of settings for a broad range of problems. In general, however, behavioral health services help individuals, couples, and families manage their personal challenges of an emotional, behavioral or cognitive nature.

What comes to mind when you think of "mental health interpreting?" Many interpreters envision interpreting in a locked-down facility with a severely psychotic patient. In fact, the great majority of mental health services are provided in primary care settings. Nonetheless, the awareness and skills required to interpret effectively for the former are just as necessary with the latter. This article will provide a simple overview of the types of interactions for which you might interpret in behavioral health. Each has its own purpose, and understanding that purpose is key to being able to provide the most appropriate and effective interpretation.

Mental health in primary care

Of all health care providers, primary care providers (PCPs) are the ones who most often identify behavioral health problems. Whether during a routine physical exam or during treatment for some other health issue, a patient's emotional or behavioral difficulties may emerge in the medical interview. As patient may introduce these concerns only obliquely, referring to them in passing or minimizing their importance, it is important that interpreters be complete and accurate in their interpretation, assuring that the provider picks up on these nuanced communications.

PCPs in turn may refer the patient to a Behavioral Health Practitioner or, depending on the problem, may treat the patient directly. For example, anti-depressants are among the most commonly prescribed medications in the U.S. at this time, most often prescribed in primary care.

An intake interview at an outpatient clinic

The first appointment at a mental health outpatient clinic is called an in-take interview. The goal of this interview is to assess the nature, range, and intensity of a patient's concerns or difficulties and to suggest a course of action: some form of therapy, medication, or referral. If counseling is identified as the appropriate response, the counselor will work with the patient to set goals, timelines and limits for the treatment.

Informal counseling

A great deal of informal counseling goes on in health care outside of what one would normally consider "behavioral health services." For example, the chaplain who stops by to visit a critically ill patient in the hospital, bringing a listening ear that helps the patient resolve a personal dilemma, is providing a mental health service. Interpreting well for this sort of informal encounter is equally important as interpreting well in a more formal treatment setting.

Formal psychotherapy

Formal counseling, or psychotherapy, may have a variety of goals: to help the patient reach a clear understanding of confusing feelings, to help a patient change unwanted behaviors, to help a patient deal better with a difficult situation. There are many different schools of thought as to how to best help patients with emotional or behavioral problems, so therapy will differ depending on patient and provider perhaps more than medical treatment does.

A key point for interpreters to remember is that it may be harder to maintain a professional distance when interpreting in psychotherapy than, for example, when interpreting in dermatology. Interpreters must be constantly aware of how they are being affected by both the content and form of the therapy, seek help if they are being negatively impacted, and remove themselves if they are unable to continue interpreting accurately and completely.

Support group

Support groups involve counseling in a group setting. For interpreters, this means being present in person to provide a linguistic bridge between (usually) one LEP member and the rest of an English-speaking group. To provide effective interpreting in this setting, interpreters must be able to perform *chuchutage* (whispered simultaneous interpreting) for the LEP member as English-speakers talk, as well as consecutive interpreting to convey the LEP member's thoughts to the group.

Drug or alcohol rehabilitation

Rehab for substance abuse can include a combination of medical and psychological treatment. Interpreting for these sessions usually requires a good deal of specific vocabulary.

Crisis intervention

Interpreting for crisis intervention can take place in person, but it is more common over the telephone. The call may come through a "911" service or through help lines set up for specific target situations or groups (rape crisis lines, teen suicide lines, domestic violence support lines, etc.) The purpose of these interactions is rapid intervention to help someone who is at immediate risk. As such, the interpreter may find a combination of emotional evaluation/support and very concrete logistical issues being discussed. It may be difficult to hear and/or understand the LEP speaker, but speed is of the essence when interpreting on these calls.

Psychiatric evaluation

A psychiatric evaluation is an assessment of a person's mental, social, and psychological functioning that often takes place when a patient first comes into contact with a given mental health facility. Patients may come referred through the Emergency Department, though the judicial system, from a Primary Care setting, or they may be brought by friends or family. The purpose of the evaluation is to get a sense of what the patient's main issues may be in order to refer the patient to the appropriate inpatient or outpatient care. In particular, providers will be evaluating the patient's mental state and whether he poses a viable threat to himself or to others. A psychiatric evaluation is not meant to constitute treatment, but simply lead to a decision about where to most appropriately refer the patient for treatment.

Family consults

A family consult in behavioral health services is much like a family consult in a medical setting. The providers' purpose in these meetings is to explain a diagnosis and discuss a treatment plan for a patient who may not be able to make decisions for himself. For interpreters, this may mean some simultaneous interpreting and the challenge of managing many people trying to talk at once. Unlike sessions directly with the patient, providers are more likely to use technical psychiatric terminology to discuss a diagnosis and treatment plan, providing interpreting challenges of both register and equivalence. The final challenge is the stigma attached to behavioral health problems in many cultures, creating a tense and sometimes adversarial environment in which to interpret.

Psychopharmacological consults

A psychopharmacological consult deals with adjusting a patient's medications. This is very similar to any medical consult with the same purpose, except that the symptoms being discussed and evaluated are both physical and psychological. Attention to correct interpreting of dosages is absolutely critical here, as even tiny changes in the dose of psychodynamic medications can lead to huge changes in a patient's functioning.

Commitment proceedings

Patients can be hospitalized for mental health treatment under two conditions. Patients can admit themselves to a psychiatric facility if they and their provider agree that in-patient treatment would be helpful. If patients are deemed to be a threat to themselves or others, however, a patient can be hospitalized against his will; this is called involuntary commitment. The process of committing a patient this way is a legal proceeding and should be treated as such by the interpreter.

Forensic evaluation

Forensic evaluations serve either to determine whether a person is psychologically fit to stand trial, or to determine the emotional state of a person during the commission of a crime. There is no therapeutic goal for this type of interview, and from an interpreter's point of view, it should be approached as an adversarial interaction, as its results will be subject to challenge in court.

These are some of the circumstances in which may be providing "mental health interpreting." As you can see, they represent a wide variety of venues, with different goals, techniques and vocabulary. The ability to adjust to these variations is the hallmark of a good mental health interpreter and will be discussed further in parts II and III of this series.

May, 2008

20.

Behavioral Health Interpreting – Part II

In Part I of this series on interpreting in behavioral health settings, I gave an overview of the various venues in which behavioral health issues are discussed. At times, interpreting for these encounters is just like other medical interpreting. However, depending on the venue, the type of health problem, and the purpose of the interview, some interpretations require a strategic shift in technique to keep all parties safe and to help further the goals of the encounter. The more you understand of what to expect in a mental health interview, the more at ease you will be and the better you will interpret.

What's the doctor looking and listening for?

In a behavioral health encounter, the provider is watching and listening for a variety of clues as to 1) the patient's orientation, 2) the patient's cognitive organization, and 3) the patient's emotional state. In particular, providers look for the following types of cues.

- **Visual cues**
  The provider notices the patient's appearance: is he clean? Are his clothes appropriate to the weather? Are there noticeable scars or wounds? The provider is also noticing the patient's motor behavior. He looks for tics (continuous involuntary movements), for nervous

habits, and for any other physical movement that might be out of the ordinary.

Implications for interpreters:
None in particular. (Of course, visual cues are not available to the phone interpreter.)

- **Orientation**
  Does the patient know **who** he is? **Where** he is? **What** day it is? Does the patient have a sense of himself within time and space and awareness of himself as a person?

  Implications for interpreters:
  Don't be surprised by questions like, "Do you know who I am? Do you know who you are? Do you know where you are? Do you know what day it is today?" Interpret just what was said. Don't help the patient to respond; don't coach the patient. If there are pauses or uncertainty in the patient's response, make sure these are communicated in your interpretation.

- **Mood and affect**
  What is the **range** of the patient's emotions? Is he appropriately happy and sad, frustrated, angry or frightened? Or is he overly emotional about something very minor? Or is there no emotional reaction at all when telling about something that would normally provoke strong feelings? (This latter is called "flat affect.") The provider will also be interested in the **intensity** of the patient's emotions, or rather, how strongly the patient feels about any given topic, and in the **stability** of those emotions. Finally, the provider is looking for **relatedness:** to what degree do the patient's emotions appropriately match what the patient is talking about?

  Implications for interpreters:
  Again, the focus for interpreters must be accuracy, to both content and tone of voice in the response. If a patient's mood swings wildly from happy to sad, from frightened to angry, this must be reflected in the interpretation. Even small nuances of change in tone signaling changes in mood must be interpreted so they will be understood.

  Another very delicate consequence for interpreters may be the need to point out if the patient's emotions seem inappropriate to the dominant society but are culturally appropriate within the patient's community. An example might be a very muted response to a terrible tragedy – or a very expansive response – that is seen as out of the norm in the dominant community but is appropriate in other cultural communities. Of course, if you feel it is appropriate to act as a culture broker it is important to make general statements only about common cultural traits, not specific statements about a patient, as we can never know what is true for a specific individual.

- **Speech and thought process and content**

  Mental health providers listen carefully to *how* patients talk in addition to what they say. What is the rate of speech -- very fast or very slow? What particular words did the patient choose to describe something? Is the same word being used over and over? Are some of the word choices unusual? Does the patient "accidentally" substitute one word for another repeatedly? Or is the patient speaking with disconnected words that don't relate to each other at all (called a "word salad")? All these are clues for the provider about possible emotional, cognitive or even organic (physical) problems.

  Providers are also paying attention to how the patient links thoughts together. Do the patient's thoughts flow logically, or do they jump all over? Does the patient go off on a tangent? Does the patient link sentences that have no relationship? Does he or she repeat certain phrases over and over? All of these are symptomatic of different diagnoses in mental health.

  Implications for interpreters:
  It is hard enough for the interpreter to reflect the pace of speech, the repetition of certain words, even the errors in word choice. An even greater challenge may come when the patient's speech makes no sense. As interpreters, we usually listen to a message, understand it, and recreate that meaning in a second language and cultural framework. What should we do when the message has no meaning? In this case, you can see how important it is to recreate the actual pattern of speech, so that the provider can perceive the symptom in the pattern. This is an advanced skill. At times it may be necessary for the interpreter simply to stop and say, "The interpreter would like to note that the patient's speech doesn't make any sense."

- **Thought process relating to cognitive functioning**
  Cognitive functioning is another area that mental health providers assess. Is the patient having delusions, i.e. perceiving the world in a way that is not based in reality? Is he or she having hallucinations, seeing or hearing things, people or voices that are not really there? Estimating the patient's grasp of reality is an important part of the evaluation and will have a key impact on the resulting treatment plan.

  Implications for interpreters:
  One of the difficulties with assessing a patient's cognitive functioning is that things like delusional thinking and hallucinations may be culturally based. For example, a Vietnamese patient may speak about being "visited" by a relative who is deceased. The patient insists this is not a dream. Is the patient hallucinating? Or is this a culture-specific experience that does not represent delusional thinking at all? In the same way, a Hispanic patient might talk about being sick because of being the victim of witchcraft. Is this delusional thinking if a belief in witchcraft is common in the patient's culture?

  As interpreters, we may need to be particularly careful to make sure that the mental health provider understands when a patient's utterance reflects a cultural view or belief that may not be shared by the dominant culture. The Vietnamese patient described above may be hallucinating, and the Hispanic patient delusional, but it is important that the provider have a cultural reference point to start from before arriving at that conclusion.

Conclusion

This article gives you a sense of what behavioral health professionals are looking and listening for, and how this impacts the interpretation. In next month's bulletin, I'll discuss some additional changes interpreters may have to make to their routine protocols in order to adapt them to mental health settings.

June, 2008

21.

Behavioral Health Interpreting – Part III

If you've read parts I and II of this series on interpreting in behavioral health venues, you've learned what sort of encounters you may be seeing and what the provider may be looking for in the patient. Part III will help you understand more about what sort of speech to prepare for in such encounters.

What sort of questions will be asked?

Mental health providers take care in phrasing their questions. As a rule, they try not to ask leading questions that point a patient toward a single "right" answer. They may use closed-ended questions for particular reasons; however, you'll often hear mental health providers (and primary care physicians as well) purposefully ask open-ended questions. These questions are phrased in such a way as to elicit a story, with no clues from the provider as to a "correct" answer.

Leading question: "You're upset, aren't you?" (Clearly, the provider thinks so.)

Closed-ended question: "Are you upset?" (Yes/no)

Open-ended question: "Tell me how you're feeling right now." (Elicits a story.)

In addition, you may hear providers respond to patients by saying "hmm" or "I see" or nothing at all. These non-committal responses are geared to encourage the patient to say more.

Implications for interpreters:

Some languages have a tendency to use more leading questions or closed-ended questions simply as a common style of speech. However, it is important that, when you interpret, you do not turn a provider's closed-ended question in to a leading question. And it is especially important that you phrase open-ended questions in English as open-ended questions in the non-English language. The provider has phrased the question that way on purpose, and the purpose must be respected in the interpretation.

If the provider is responding with sounds like "hmm" or simple silence, fight the urge to fill the silence. The provider is using the silence as a means of encouraging the patient to keep talking.

When should other techniques be changed?

There are a few other times when interpreters may have to adapt techniques commonly used in medical interpreting.

- If possible, do an expanded pre-session. Unlike medical interpreting, with its short sessions and hurried providers, behavioral health sessions tend to be longer and providers more willing to conduct a pre-session with the interpreter. You need to ask about the purpose of the encounter, what you can expect in terms of the patient's behavior, and any special issues the provider thinks you should know about. This information will help you be better prepared and do a better interpretation.

- Adjust your positioning according to the situation. Under certain conditions, it may be inappropriate or unsafe to position yourself as you normally do in medical settings. A paranoid patient might feel anxious to have you beside and bit behind him; a violent patient might need to be given more space. Discuss positioning with the behavioral health professional and respect any guidance you are given.

- Be prepared to switch to simultaneous mode. Patients who are traumatized may have difficulty telling their story. If they finally do begin to share, asking them to pause to let you interpret may shut them down again. This is one of those times when it may be best to move closer to the provider and switch to a soft simultaneous interpreting.

- Watch out for transference and counter-transference. Patients sometimes work out their problems in other relationships through their relationship with their therapist; for example, a patient who is angry with his spouse yells at the therapist instead. This is called transference. Patients can transfer emotions onto interpreters as well. If you find the patient expressing strong emotions toward you - either positive or negative - that seem to have no reasonable basis, consider that these feelings likely have nothing to do with you as an individual at all. Therefore it is best not to take anything that the patient says or does personally.

  In a reverse situation, therapists can sometimes find themselves working out their own issues through their relationship with a patient. This is called counter-transference, and this is poor practice. Again, it can happen to interpreters as well. If you find yourself strongly attracted to a patient, wanting to take care of a patient, or particularly angry with a patient, you may need to ask yourself why. Talk to the therapist if you have to; keeping clear boundaries in these cases is especially important.

Take care of yourself.

Interpreters working in behavioral health can be exposed to all sorts of awful stuff that patients talk about. Interpreters can be **retraumatized** by hearing a patient recount terrible experiences that may have been shared by the interpreter as well. Or they can experience **vicarious trauma** simply by having to listen to some of the things that human beings do to each other. In some ways, the act of first-person interpreting, in which the interpreter speaks with the patient's voice (for example, "I was raped.") can be especially devastating.

Unfortunately, because good interpreters are typically so successful at being invisible, providers often forget to consider how the interpretation may have affected the interpreter. Be aware if a session has impacted you deeply - if you feel extraordinarily sad, if you start having nightmares, if your eating or sleeping patterns change. Finding someone with whom to debrief often helps, whether this is your supervisor, a member of the clergy, a mental health provider or a colleague. Be sure, of course, not to release any information that could identify the patient, but do find a place to discuss your experience in the interpretation. After all, you are a valuable resource in language access, and we want you to stay healthy!

If medical interpreting is just emerging as a profession, mental health interpreting is still in its infancy. Though one of the more difficult venues in which to provide interpreting services, it is also one of the least developed as well. Indeed, the experiences of your generation of pioneer mental health interpreters will be those that form the basis for the protocols in this field in the future.

July 2008

22.

Interpreting at the End of Life – Part I

Interpreting for patients, their families, and their care providers at the end of life is a delicate and important undertaking. This is the first of two articles focusing on interpreting for patients at the end of their lives. This one will deal with what to expect. The better prepared you are--intellectually and emotionally--to deal with these challenges, the better the quality of care you can provide.

How has end-of-life care changed?

Advances in medical care have made a profound change in end-of-life care in the U.S. Unlike earlier times when infectious disease and physical trauma were the preeminent killers and when death took place relatively rapidly at home or at the site of the trauma, most Americans today die of chronic illnesses such as cardiac disease and cancer, and most die in institutions. As a result, many Americans have never seen a person die, never seen a dead body and are not prepared to talk about death.

Medical advances have changed how we experience death in the U.S. in another way. Technical life support (such as respirators and feeding tubes) has advanced to the point that critically ill patients can often be kept alive through the use of artificial means, even without the hope of meaningful recovery. But who decides if a patient stays on artificial life support or is allowed to die? Remember that the dominant culture in this country holds the rights of the individual in highest regard. Therefore, a number of legal protections have been put in place to assure that decisions of this nature are made with respect for the patient's own wishes, even if the patient is not capable of expressing those wishes him- or herself at the time a decision needs to be made. Two of these protections are the Advance Directive and the Health Proxy.

Advance Directive (Living Will)

An Advance Directive is a legal document in which the patient specifies beforehand what sort of emergency measures should be taken if he or she is not in condition to make a decision at the time. Advance Directives usually deal with 1) whether the patient wants to receive CPR and defibrillation if the heart stops, 2) whether a patient wants to be put on a respirator if pulmonary function declines, and 3) whether a patient want a feeding tube inserted if he or she can no longer eat. An Advance Directive should be registered in the patient's chart and can be changed by the patient at any time.

Durable Power of Attorney for Health Care (Health Proxy)

A Durable Power of Attorney for Health Care or a Health Proxy is a legal document that names an individual who has the right to make health decisions on behalf of the patient if the patient is unable to communicate his or her own decisions. These documents also reside in the patient's medical record and can also be changed by the patient at any time. If neither an Advance Directive nor a Health Proxy is on file, and if the patient cannot make his decisions known, healthcare providers will turn to the next of kin to make these decisions. This is so even if the next of kin is not the person closest to the patient or most likely to know his wishes.

Do-Not-Resuscitate Order

If requested in the Advance Directive or dictated by the Health Proxy, a doctor may write a Do-Not-Resuscitate order (DNR). A DNR means that no extraordinary measures will be taken to revive the patient if the heart stops. Rather, the patient will be allowed to die.

Organ Donation form

A patient's willingness to donate his or her organs for transplant can be noted on the driver's license and/or in the patient record. This tremendous act of compassion will allow the patient's otherwise healthy corneas, heart, lungs, liver, and kidneys to be harvested soon after the patient's death so that they can be transplanted into patients who would otherwise die. While these documents become especially important at the end of life, most hospitals ask about Advance Directives, Health Proxies and organ donation with every patient who is admitted. Even patients admitted for routine procedures will be asked to fill out an Advance Directive. This request often surprises and dismays relatively healthy patients who, if not familiar with this practice, may see it as an indication that the provider expects them to die.

Changes in discussing end of life issues

In comparison with healthcare providers in many parts of the world, providers in the U.S. are fairly open in talking about end-of-life issues. The underlying motivation for this is a strong conviction that patients have a right to know what is happening to them and that participating in making decisions that affect their care will lead to a more peaceful death.

Family will usually be brought into these discussions, unless the patient specifically chooses otherwise. The goals of treatment will be discussed: whether to treat the disease, to extend life as long as possible even if a cure is not possible, to improve the quality of the life remaining by controlling symptoms, or simply to keep the patient comfortable as the disease runs its natural course.

Patients and families may be offered the option of hospice care. Hospice is an approach to caring for patients at the end of their lives that approaches death as a natural process. Hospice care, which can be provided in a nursing facility or at home, helps maintain the patient pain-free with the highest possible quality of life until the end. In order to get hospice services, the patient must sign a release recognizing that he has six months or less to live and forgoing any curative treatment.

Many hospitals and hospice programs also offer support programs for families of patients. Specifically, family support services will help the family members organize their loved one's care, and bereavement counseling to help family members deal with their grief may be offered even before the patient dies.

Comfort care (palliative care)

When nothing more can be done to cure the patient or the patient chooses to end curative treatments, the patient will be given comfort care, also called palliative care. The goal of this care is to keep the patient as comfortable as possible, so that he or she will not suffer as death approaches. Comfort care includes the removal of monitors, the use of very strong pain medication, fever control, prevention of bed sores, etc, but does not attempt to treat the root cause of illness.

Active dying

At the very end, the patient will enter into the stage called "active dying." During this stage the patient may become more withdrawn and confused, disinterested in eating or drinking, incontinent, cool to the touch and bluish in color. Breathing will become irregular and shallow, alternating between rapid and slow, and intermixed with rattling or gurgling sounds. These are all natural results of body systems shutting down. The process will end when the heart stops.

Interpreting during a code

If a DNR is in place, nothing will be done when the heart stops. However, if no DNR order has been registered, the first clinical staff person who perceives the heart stoppage will "call a code" (also called "Code Blue" or "Code 119"; each institution is different). A score of clinicians will come running: all the nurses on the floor, the head resident, the attending, an anesthesiologist, a cardiologist, etc. Cardiopulmonary resuscitation (CPR) will be started immediately until a crash cart arrives, at which point a defibrillator will be used to try to restart the patient's heart. An airway may be inserted and multiple medications added via IV. The scene will appear chaotic, but in truth, this is a carefully choreographed dance in which each individual has a part to play.

As an interpreter, your part is to 1) stay calm, 2) get yourself and any family members out of the clinicians' way, even if that means getting them out of the room, 3) tell the family that the patient is having difficulty and that the staff is responding, that the apparent chaos they are seeing is normal for these circumstances, that the medical staff is doing everything it can to help their loved one and that a doctor will come talk to them as soon as possible. Do not tell them that everything will be all right, and do not try to interpret everything that is being said, as it will be too confusing.

After death

When the patient does die, it is usually a nurse who notes the time of death. A doctor will be called, who will legally pronounce the patient dead. The family will be allowed to stay with their beloved one as long as they wish, to say good-bye, at which point the remains will be removed to the morgue until the funeral home of the family's choice comes to claim them.

Even if you know what to expect during the process of dying in an American hospital, interpreting for patients at the end of life can be very difficult. In the next article in this series, I'll address some of the cultural differences that often come into play in these interactions, as well as some of the unique challenges that interpreters face.

August, 2006

23.

Interpreting at the End of Life – Part II

In Part I of this series, I addressed what to expect when interpreting for a patient who is dying. Being cognitively and emotionally prepared for what you may experience in these settings will help you stay calmer and focus on your task: that of facilitating the communication between patient, family and hospital staff. To do that well, there are a number of issues with which you will need to contend.

There are few areas of healthcare in which people depend more on the comforting familiarity of cultural patterns than around death. Unfortunately, as we know, different cultures hold differing expectations and differing definitions of acceptable behavior. Interpreters must be aware of these differences and ready to point them out if they are leading to a breakdown in communication.

One difference is the manner in which bad news should be discussed and, indeed, whether death can be discussed openly at all. As mentioned in the previous article, healthcare providers in the U.S. expect to speak fairly directly with patients about their prognosis, while this practice can be seen as shocking, inappropriate, rude, and even deadly to members of other cultures. In many places round the world, such discussions are held with family members only, and **they** decide how and how much to tell the patient. If such material is being discussed for the first time with a patient or family, and if you feel that such a discussion would be inappropriate in the family's culture, you can bring this up to the physician so that it can be discussed openly. After bringing the matter up, it is then your job to accept whatever the family and doctor decide.

Other cultural differences that arise when a patient is dying include:

The definition of family

For hospital purposes, "next of kin" means parents, siblings and children. Aunts, uncles, cousins and many of the people counted as "family" in cultures based on extended families, may not be considered as such at the hospital. This can cause unending grief unless clearly negotiated with the institution.

The spiritual needs of the patient and the family

Hospitals these days can be amazingly flexible in accommodating and supporting a patient's spiritual beliefs and cultural practices. I know of hospitals in the Central Valley of California that regularly allow traditional healing ceremonies to be conducted in Hmong patients' rooms by shamen. I know of another that temporarily disabled a smoke detector to allow sage to be burned in a Native American patient's room as part of a healing ceremony, and another that allowed the remains of a recently deceased Muslim patient to continue in the patient room much longer than normal so that the extended community could pay its respects. In order for the hospital to be responsive, however, the family must be sure to communicate their needs to the hospital staff with some prior notice. Often the hospital chaplain will play a role in helping to get these needs accommodated.

Understanding of hospice

The hospice movement was born as an alternative to the practice of keeping patients alive at all costs, even beyond the hope of a meaningful recovery. Hospice recognizes death as a natural part of life, allowing patients to spend their last days with dignity, without pain, and surrounded by those they love. Ironically, to families unfamiliar with the implications of unquestioned life support, offering to place a patient in hospice can seem like a slap in the face. Families offered hospice can view this as a sign of racism, of classism, of anti-immigrant sentiment – as a sign that the medical staff is sending the patient home to die because they could not be bothered to take all possible steps to save her. To the contrary, hospice is a program steeped in respect for the patient and his or her family, based on a recognition that, for this patient at this time, hospital care will not stave off death but simply make the patient more miserable.

The symbolic meaning related to the removal of life support

What decision could be harder for a family than whether or not to remove life support from a loved one? Providers often see this as primarily a question of the family coming to terms with letting go of a patient who will not get better. However, depending on the family's religious beliefs, removal of life support can be seen as hurting the patient's spiritual well being (by artificially ending a life while there are still spiritual lessons to be learned) or as hurting the decision-maker's spiritual well-being (by making him a murderer). It can be seen as showing disrespect to the patient by not doing "everything possible" to save her, or as showing disrespect to God by not seeing His hand in the technology that is keeping the patient alive. It is crucial that providers understand what this decision **means** to the family in order to help counsel them through it.

How human remains should be cared for

Different cultures have different norms for handling human remains. As discussed earlier, when a person dies in a hospital in the U.S., the body will be detached from any IV lines or monitors, and the family will be given time with the deceased to say good-bye. The body will then be covered and taken to the morgue, often at night when other patients are asleep, where it will stay until it is picked up by a funeral home (mortuary). If the family needs other arrangements to be made (e.g. extended visitation, purification rituals etc.) they must discuss it with the hospital staff, preferably before the death occurs.

In addition to being aware of cultural differences that may lead to misunderstandings, there are a number of other challenges that interpreters face when interpreting at the end of life. For example, in both languages you may find that people use a peculiar oblique vocabulary when talking about death. In English, you will hear phrases like, "when she passes over," "when she moves on," "when the time comes," "as she fades," "when she goes to her rest," "when she goes to that better place." Other languages have equally indirect ways of talking about dying. In choosing the equivalents you use when interpreting, your challenge is to respect the softer, veiled nature of this speech, while making sure that the meaning behind it is understood. For example, the doctor may feel that by talking about "comfort care" he has made it clear that he can do nothing more to save the patient's life, while that code word may mean nothing to the family. It is important that the family understand that the provider is indeed talking about death.

Another challenge as an interpreter is accommodating the spiritual beliefs of the patient, when they are beliefs you do not share. The challenge can be emotional, as it may mean interpreting prayers that you do not believe, interpreting rituals that you do not recognize, interpreting for spiritual leaders you do not respect. The challenge can also be linguistic, as you may not be familiar with the frozen register required in some prayers and rituals. One way or the other, interpreting in these situations is part of your work as a professional interpreter.

The physical environment surrounding a dying patient can also take some getting used to. There are smells and sounds and sights you may not have experienced before. Talking to hospital staff about what to expect before going into an encounter can help, as will simply gaining experience.

The greatest challenge in interpreting at the end of life lies in dealing with the feelings that such interpreting will elicit within you. How do you see death? Does this interpreting make you think about the eventual deaths of those you love, remember the death of someone close to you, confront the inevitability of your own death? Do you find yourself grieving for the passing of patients for whom you have interpreted often, or even for patients whom you barely knew? All of this is normal and common and **must not be simply ignored**. Make sure you have someone to talk to about these feelings and thoughts. The hospital chaplain, who is specially trained in this sort of counseling, is a good resource, as are other members of the treating team. Doctors and nurses in oncology, in transplant units, and in intensive care units will have ample experience with these challenges.

As an interpreter, facilitating communication between patients, families and care providers at life's end can be both a responsibility and a blessing. It is not the same as interpreting for a blood draw or an eye exam or a primary care visit. As important as these are, interpreting well at the end of life is a special skill, a combination of technical knowledge, insight and compassion. Some interpreters consider it a privilege to be present as another human being passes from this reality to another, while others view it as a service, and still others feel it only as a burden. Whatever your personal feelings, the facilitation of clear communication at such a difficult time is, without doubt, a gift to dying patients, their families and the providers who care for them.

September, 2006

24.

Interpreting Prayer

In September of 2006, a question was posted to the listserv of the National Council on Interpreting in Health Care that set off a flurry of interesting discussion. It had to do with interpreting prayer.

Imagine being called to interpret at a hospital. Instead of a doctor, you find that the provider for whom you are interpreting is a chaplain - or a pastor or a priest or a rabbi or a mullah or other religious leader. At the patient's request, the chaplain offers a prayer. It is a prayer from a religion you do not espouse. There are things in it you don't believe. Even worse, it is a prayer that has a fixed form — in any language — and you do not know that fixed form. What should you do?

The same difficulty can arise from the chaplain reading from sacred texts, or from the vocabulary the chaplain uses to talk to the patient about spiritual matters. There are two delicate matters here for interpreters. One is ethical and the other linguistic. Let's tackle the ethical problem first.

There are few things human beings hold closer to their hearts than their religious beliefs. Therefore, it can be very challenging for an interpreter to interpret prayer, or sacred text, or conversations about God that reflect beliefs that the interpreter does not share. If you find yourself in such a position, how can you handle it? Here are some suggestions that may help.[14]

[14] All quotes and references in this article appeared on the NCIHC listserv discussion of September 2006 and are included here with permission.

1. **Be aware that spiritual support is now considered an integral part of healing.**
   Don't be surprised if you are asked to interpret visits between the patient and the hospital chaplain. If we are to consider ourselves professional healthcare interpreters, we must be willing to interpret for all venues in healthcare, and that includes spiritual care.

2. **Remember your role.**
   Your purpose as an interpreter is to facilitate understanding in communication between people who are speaking different languages. The content of the speech is not your concern - only the rendering of it in such a way as to communicate clearly the meaning. Just like when interpreting cultural beliefs that you do not share or medical advice that you think is ridiculous, professional interpreters keep their opinions about the content to be interpreted to themselves. Frankly, within this setting and on this subject, your opinion doesn't count.

3. **Remember that you are not the speaker.**
   Keep in mind that this speech is not coming from you; it is coming from the speaker. The words are not meant to be, nor are they understood to be, a reflection of your beliefs. You are only the means of communication, not the source of the message.

4. **You can withdraw if you can't do a good job.**
   If the content to be interpreted bothers you so much that you simply can't interpret accurately, you can always withdraw. Withdrawal of the interpreter, of course, causes a major disruption for the provider and patient. If you withdraw too often, then, be prepared to not be called to interpret as often.

There is another difficulty regarding interpreting prayer and sacred text, however. While some prayers are offered in a free form, rather like a conversation with God, others are written in a certain way, using specific language that cannot be changed. This is called "frozen register." Two good examples of "frozen register" from Christian religious practice are The Lord's Prayer and the Rosary. "Our Father in heaven, may Your name be thought of as holy" is just not the same thing as "Our Father, who art in heaven, hallowed by Thy name." Unlike other interpreting work, a meaning-for-meaning interpretation is not good enough; the interpretation must follow the prescribed words used in the prayer. This is true for the interpretation of sacred text as well.

So what is an interpreter to do? You cannot be expected to know by heart the official translations of all the world's sacred texts in your interpreted languages. Neither is misinterpreting somebody's beloved revealed prayers an option. Here are some useful suggestions, then, offered by interpreters through the NCIHC listserv:

- If you know ahead of time that you will be interpreting prayers, you can do some prior research. Juan Gutierrez from Kentucky points out that the Catholic Church has issued official versions of the common prayers in different languages, some of which can be found online. For Spanish, you can go to http://www.catholic.org/clife/prayers. This is true for a number of other faiths as well, among them the Church of Jesus Christ of Latter Day Saints (http://www.lds.org/gospellibrary/0,5082,4-1,00.html), the Jehovah's Witnesses (http://www.watchtower.org/languages.htm), and the Bahá'í Faith (http://www.bahaiprayers.org). Of course, such resources are useful only if you know ahead of time what prayers you will need.

- Mark Bowers of Saint Francis Memorial Hospital suggests asking the chaplain if a prayer is a "rote prayer" (that is, if it is recited in frozen register). If it is, he simply asks the patient if he or she would like to recite the prayer together with the chaplain. Then, as Mark puts it, "I don't need to say anything; they speak in English and Spanish, (and) I get to marvel over how people translate poetry." Mark also mentioned that his hospital has put in a stock of Spanish-language Bibles both so that interpreters can read directly from the translated texts and so that patients can take the Bibles with them.

- A final approach is to simply admit to patient and provider that you are not familiar with the prayers or texts being interpreted, and to ask for patience and assistance in interpreting them correctly. Please note, this is not an invitation to share your own religious affiliation or your own religious beliefs; that is never appropriate within a professional interpreting environment. An admission of ignorance, however, will at least assure the patient that any misinterpretations are not meant as disrespect.

We talk a lot in healthcare interpreting about learning the technical vocabulary of cardiology and oncology and pediatrics. We discuss the ethical difficulties of interpreting foul language, lies and other content with which we feel uncomfortable. Interpreting religious content is no different: it has its own special vocabulary and requires the same commitment to be non-judgmental, accurate, complete and appropriate. And it is just as important for the patient's well being. Indeed, the only thing I can think of that's better than helping patients to heal physically might just be to help them heal spiritually.

October, 2006

Section 3

The Under-appreciated Interpreter

25.

My Daughter Speaks English – Why are YOU Here?

Have you ever interpreted in the following scenario?

You report in to interpret on-site. The MA calls your patient's name, and when you step up to introduce yourself, your patient says, "My daughter here speaks English, so I don't need an interpreter."

Or how about this?

You take a call to interpret over the phone. You greet the provider, greet the patient, and the session starts. The doctor asks a question, and before you can interpret, a voice answers. In English.

Or this one –

You are interpreting over the phone for a doctor and a family. So far, the patient has waited for your interpretation and answered in her non-English language. But suddenly, another voice starts asking questions in English. The doctor responds without waiting for you to interpret. The doctor and English speaker get into a long discussion. Without you. And more importantly, without the patient.

What a mess! What to do? How to manage all these interactions? The presence of an

English speaker in an interpreted session can cause real confusion, especially if the provider is not skilled in negotiating a bilingual conversation. It may be up to you to find a way through. Here are some suggestions to try out:

Problem: The patient declines your services, as an English-speaking family member has come to interpret.

Recommendation: Make sure the patient understands that 1) you are a trained professional healthcare interpreter, and 2) the patient will not be charged for your services. Assure the patient that his or her family members are welcome to attend the medical appointment as well; they have an important role to play in providing support, so they shouldn't have to be burdened with having to interpret as well. If the patient still declines your services, explain the situation to the medical center staff and ask them what they would like you to do. Many facilities have their own policies regarding these circumstances. Most of all, stay calm, stay friendly, and stay professional.

Problem: The English-speaking family member starts to answer for the patient.

Recommendation: While it is inappropriate for the family member to answer for the patient, let the provider handle that issue. Your concern is to make sure that the patient understands what the family member is saying. If you are interpreting in person, move next to the patient and provide a simultaneous interpretation of the English conversation to the patient. If you are interpreting over the phone, your best bet is to start taking careful notes of the conversation. The next time a question is directed to the patient and you get a chance to interpret, tell the provider that you will quickly summarize the English discussion that just went on and then ask his question. Then do just that.

Problem: The English-speaking family member and the doctor get into an English conversation from which the patient is excluded.

Recommendation: Again, your concern as the interpreter is to assure that everyone in the room understands everything that is being said. The same techniques mentioned above work in this situation as well. You just may have to take notes for a longer time.

Problem: The English-speaking family member claims that you are misinterpreting.

Recommendation: As hard as it may be, don't get defensive. If the family challenges your interpretation (e.g." That's not what she said!"), ask for the patient or provider to repeat what had been said and interpret it again. If the English-speaker accuses you of misinterpreting and offers an alternative interpretation that you feel is dangerously inaccurate, ask the provider to clarify with the patient. Don't get caught up in defending your interpretation, justifying your mistakes, making excuses, or apologizing. Any of these things can distract from the purpose of the interaction: the patient's healthcare.

Problem: The patient speaks a little English and goes back and forth between English and the non-English language. ARGH! This is the worst! You can't get into any kind of interpreting rhythm under these circumstances, and it's hard to know what the patient understands of the English speech and what needs to be interpreted. In addition, since the patient's English is lacking, it's also hard to know what the provider understands of what the patient says.

Recommendation: First, try to interpret only the parts of the speech that were expressed in the non-English language. You may have to repeat some of the English speech in order to make the message intelligible. If things get too confusing, you may have to ask the provider to suggest to the patient that it would be better for the clarity of the communication if he would speak only in one language or the other.

Conclusion

I'm sure there are other permutations of the frustrating mixture of languages. Just remember, if you were there with your LEP family member, you would want to intervene too. As the interpreter, just keep your focus on making sure that everyone is understanding; stay calm, stay detached and stay professional. And stifle that secret wish that the English-speaking daughter would just stay in the waiting room; you're there for the patient, but she's there for her Mom.

September 2008

26.

Target Practice is Fun (Unless You're the Target)

or How to Handle Angry Clients

For all that healthcare and social service encounters should be collaborative interactions, they can also contain conflict. The provider gets frustrated with the patient. The patient gets angry at the provider. You interpret the anger both ways, and let the speakers work the problem out.

However, there are the times when a speaker chooses to focus his or her frustration not on the other speaker or on a frustrating situation itself, but on you. And other than being the facilitator of communication, you have suddenly become a target. Has this ever happened to you?

- The patient questions your ability and calls you "stupid."
- The speakerphone is of poor quality, or there is background noise, or the speaker is mumbling, making it difficult to hear and understand.
- The provider gets impatient as you ask for repeats.
- The patient does not answer the provider's questions, and the provider holds you responsible.
- You accurately interpret a rude comment or an angry tone of voice,

and the listener blames you for what was said.

- Speaker #1 will not comply with what Speaker #2 wants. Speaker #2 does not get angry at Speaker #1; Speaker #2 gets angry at you.

Doesn't this just drive you crazy? It's not fair, it's not your fault, and it can even make you consider a career change. But before you turn in your ID, be assured that you can handle these situations. Here's how.

Rule #1: Stay calm.

This is also Rule #2-10, which gives you an idea of how important it is! Losing your temper, for any reason, only makes you look unprofessional and fuels the fire of the person who is frustrated or upset. It will not help resolve the situation. So, no matter how greatly you are provoked, no matter how offensive or unjust the attack, no matter how justified a cutting response would be, you must remain detached and calm. Taking deep breaths helps.

Rule #11: Be unfailingly polite.

You can throw darts at a picture of your client when you hang up or get home. While you're working, you must maintain a polite tone of voice and use polite language, no matter what.

Rule #12: If blamed for the content of the speaker's message, clarify your role.

Sad but true - there are still many people, both English speaking and LEP, who do not know what an interpreter's work entails. If Speaker #1 refuses to comply with a request from Speaker #2 (or says something angry or sidesteps a question) and Speaker #2 honestly believes that this is coming from you, it is understandable that you become the target for some frustration. When challenged, a useful response is: "The interpreter is interpreting exactly what __________ said." Stop there. You don't need to say any more.

Rule #13: If challenged about the quality of the interpretation, be honest.

If you are sure that your interpretation was correct, you might respond: "The interpreter is interpreting exactly what the patient is saying." If there is a possibility that your interpretation might be in error, a better response would be: "The interpreter will check again."

Rule #14: If the speaker's comments to you are offensive, ignore it if at all possible.

'D-TIP' is the rule: Don't Take It Personally. Remember, most people who create conflict are frustrated with themselves, with the situation, or with the person with whom they are conversing. They are simply taking it out on you because you're the only one in the interaction who can understand them.

Rule #15: Stay transparent.

Some interpreter trainers counsel that any comment directed at you, no matter how angry, should just be interpreted on as if it were directed to the listener, even if it is clear that it was directed to you. In my experience, this is a guaranteed way of making an angry speaker even angrier, and it does nothing to resolve the situation. However, when you do respond to a comment that has been directed to you, remember to give your listener a quick summary of what is being discussed, e.g. "The doctor has asked me why you don't answer her question. I'm going to suggest she ask you." If you are not transparent, listeners will certainly pick up on conflict in the tone of voice anyway, and this can be very stressful if the listener doesn't know the nature of or reason for the conflict.

Rule #16: Use assertive communication.

When communicating assertively, you start from a position of respect for both yourself and your listener. You recognize the listener's concern, and then you go on to clearly state your own needs in the matter. So, for example, let's say that you are interpreting over the phone, and that poor technology is making it hard to hear. You ask the patient and provider to speak up several times. Finally, the doctor says in frustration, "Interpreter, what's wrong with you, are you deaf?" You might say "I apologize for the interruptions, I am having trouble hearing on the speakerphone because of the background noise, and I want to do as accurate an interpretation as possible. It might help if both you and the patient moved closer to the speakerphone, or if the background noise could be controlled."

Rule #17: You can always offer to withdraw.

If the conflict is getting in the way of the encounter continuing, you might do best to offer to withdraw. At the very least, this reminds the speakers that you are their only way to communicate with each other and can often help calm down the situation so that you can return to interpreting. If the speaker is being personally abusive to you, rather than simply expressing frustration, you are permitted to withdraw even if they don't want you to do so. Something like this might be appropriate: "I regret that I am unable to continue to interpret under these circumstances. Please call the company to obtain the services of a different interpreter." As always, save withdrawing for really extreme cases.

Rule #18: Remember that you will not necessarily be able to keep everybody happy all the time.

No matter how well you handle some situations, the client or the LEP individual may go away unhappy. They may even lodge a complaint. This doesn't necessarily mean that you didn't handle the situation well.

Rule #19: Phone home.

If you should ever experience this kind of conflict in an interpreting assignment, make sure to call your company's Quality Assurance department as soon as you can. It is better for them to hear your side of the story first in case the client calls to complain. They will be able to explain your actions to a client as long as you were behaving appropriately.

Conclusion

Being a target is certainly no fun. Getting shot hurts, and shooting back simply doesn't help. But by practicing the techniques mentioned above, you can build a professional armor around yourself that will make it easier to deal with conflictive situations constructively. Stay calm, stay professional, stay focused, and the bullets will bounce right off.

September 2003/March 2009

27.

Training the Whole Team

Imagine a soccer team with a new member who knows a fantastic new play that is guaranteed to win the World Cup. Except nobody else on the team has been taught the play. Anyone want to bet on the outcome?

As interpreters, we can often feel like that new player on the soccer team. We have a great new play that will really help further communication - but nobody else knows it! That's not going to work; for the play to be effective, the whole team needs to work together.

In fact, as the use of trained interpreters becomes more widespread, more effort is being made to teach healthcare providers to work effectively with interpreters. Getting docs into training, however, is often challenging. Most doctors work either as independent practitioners or under contract to a hospital or clinic. As such, the hospital cannot require them to take a particular training. So those of us who are coaching this team have gotten pretty resourceful about reaching this elusive audience.

Medical School

One place that physicians, nurses and social workers are now learning how to work with interpreters is in their professional training. Medical schools, nursing schools and social work schools are starting to include interpreting issues as part of their standard curriculum.

In medical schools, this material is typically introduced in the second year, as part of the coursework on medical interviewing. Classroom discussion of language access and interpreting is often complemented by including some LEP individuals as "standardized patients" with whom the medical students practice their interviewing skills. At the University of Washington, these students first practice taking a simple health history through an interpreter; in the second round, however, these LEP "patients" are prepped to present with a health problem about which they hold a traditional non-biomedical belief. Students must learn not only basic interviewing skills, but to negotiate meaning through the interpreter as well.

At the University of Rochester, the medical school annually hosts "Deaf Strong Hospital" for the first year medical students. In this role-playing exercise, volunteers from the local deaf community staff a series of clinical "stations" (pharmacy, outpatient, surgical consent, etc.) Students are given a specific disease scenario and must navigate their way through the system. No voice is allowed, only gesture or Sign if they know it. A small number of students are allowed to use interpreters. Misunderstandings abound, of course, except for those students who had interpreter services. Follow-up discussion with faculty and deaf volunteers helps students learn the importance of language access in health care, both for speakers of non-English languages as well as for the deaf.

An informal query to the NCIHC listserv in 2003 identified a number of other medical schools that also include interpreter use in their basic curriculum, including Harvard, Oregon Health and Sciences University, UCLA, Northwestern, the University of Chicago, the University of Nebraska, and the University of New Mexico Physician Assistant program. This list is growing as interpreters become a more common and accepted member of the healthcare team.

Residency programs

Residency programs present another great opportunity to teach about language access. Unlike medical students, residents are actively attending patients, so they tend to find language issues very real. And unlike staff physicians, residents are still technically students, so programs can require them to attend training. Finally, due to the complexities surrounding medical school curriculum development, it's easier to get a session on language access included into a residency program than to get it included into a medical school curriculum.

As hospitals with residency programs develop comprehensive interpreter services, the managers of these services are increasingly finding residency programs to be one venue for training the providers whom the interpreters will serve.

Grand Rounds

"Grand Rounds" started as medical students accompanying a senior physician as he or she did rounds, checking up on patients at a hospital. It was an opportunity for the more experienced doctor to teach novices based on real cases.

Nowadays, Grand Rounds can take place in a clinical setting or in a conference room, and both experienced and novice physicians attend. Since doctors routinely learn about other advances in medicine through Grand Rounds, it's an effective venue for teaching about interpreter use as well.

Brown Bag Lunches

Personally, I've never been to a "Brown Bag Lunch" where there was a brown bag in sight! Usually lunch is provided for staff, as an incentive for them to attend a presentation. Started by pharmaceutical companies as a means to introduce new medications to physicians, this strategy is now being borrowed by Interpreter Service Managers as a means of getting providers a quick 30-40 minute instruction on how to work with an interpreter.

Conferences

Did you know that in many states physicians need continuing education credits in order to keep their licenses? One way docs meet these requirements is by attending conferences. Sessions regarding interpreter use are sometimes included on the program, although they tend to be poorly attended, mostly reaching physicians who are already interested and knowledgeable on the subject.

Web-based Training

The newest way to reach physicians is over the Internet. Pressed for time and impatient with the pace of on-site trainings, many doctors are now getting their continuing education credits through web-based training programs. One such program is offered by Medical Directions at http://www.vlh.com, called *Communicating with Interpreters in Healthcare*. This 2-credit course is being purchased by hospitals for their physician staff as a means of building their skills in working with interpreters.

What can interpreters do?

If web-based training is the newest way to reach docs, the oldest way is one you learned in your basic interpreter training: the pre-session. On-site interpreters probably do more in those 30-seconds before an interpreting session to impact how well doctors work with them than all the Grand Rounds ever done. While many of us moan that we shouldn't have to be teaching doctors these basic skills, it does lead to clearer communication, and that is what we are all about.

Of course, training the physicians is great, but this is just the start. We also have to reach the nurses. And the Medical Assistants. And the front desk staff. Then there are the Physical Therapists, the Occupational Therapists, the Speech Therapists and the just plain Therapists. The PAs, the TAs and the NPs. The Social Workers, the Case Workers, the Account Reps and the Patient Reps. Phlebotomists, nutritionists. Chaplains and Child Life.

Wow. That's a big team. We better get cracking, because we have a new play that can save lives and the whole team better learn how it works.

March 2007

28.

The Docs that Drive You Crazy

I am often asked to share some techniques for dealing with "uncooperative providers." Throughout the years that I have trained interpreters, I have heard many creative ideas as to how to handle difficult docs. Some were great; some were questionable; and some were just plain illegal. We need to find some good ways of dealing with providers who make our jobs difficult, and in the process, compromise clear communication with the patient.

So here are the top ten ways in which providers can drive you to distraction and some ideas of what to do about it.

1. **They start without you.**
   What a way to begin: you arrive on time for an appointment only to discover that the provider has started without you. Of course, many providers are under great pressure to see an ever larger number of patients per day. If one patient no-shows or if the provider finishes early with another, and if they do not have a clear understanding of the critical role the interpreter plays, they may choose to move ahead with their appointments rather than to wait for the interpreter.

   What to do? In that moment, the most professional response is to knock on the exam room door, enter when invited, introduce yourself briefly to provider and patient, position yourself and calmly begin to interpret. It is unlikely the doctor will go back and start over now that you are present, so you should be extra aware of any signs that the patient has not understood what was said. After the appointment, report to your supervisor so that they can let the institution know that this provider is seeing patients without an interpreter.

2. **They assume you are the patient's son/daughter, brother/sister, caretaker, chauffeur, friend - anything but another professional.** If providers are accustomed to using family and friends to interpret, I suppose it is natural for them to assume that you are one or the other. However, it is important that you immediately clarify your role. Your dress, your demeanor, your clearly visible name badge and your calm, professional behavior should be effective clues to the provider that you are part of the healthcare team, but if not, a concise pre-session should clarify any misapprehensions.

3. **They decide they learned enough Spanish in Cuernavaca last week (or Russian in Moscow last summer, or Vietnamese in Saigon 30 years ago) that they don't need you to interpret.** This is rather like my taking a first-aid course and deciding that I can treat patients in the ER. I don't think most providers who take this attitude realize how insulting it is or the risk they run of a serious miscommunication with the patient. However, we gain nothing as interpreters in contradicting a provider or embarrassing him/her in front of the patient. An effective strategy in these cases is to offer to sit in on the appointment "just in case" a misunderstanding occurs. Keep an eye on the patient's body language, and if it appears that the provider is stumbling or the patient does not understand, simply slip into interpreting without calling attention to the fact. Non-fluent providers will inevitably slip back into their dominant language when communication in their weak second language becomes too difficult.

4. **They talk to you instead of to the patient.** This is a sure sign that the provider has never been trained to work with interpreters, and it is one problem that can be avoided by a short pre-session. If the provider still addresses you, you can help redirect the provider's attention by looking at the patient while the provider is speaking and by using a small open-handed gesture to the patient. If the behavior persists, you can intervene and ask the provider to speak directly to the patient. If the behavior still

continues, give up; any more interventions will simply create a greater barrier to communication. If possible, however, you might want to talk to the provider after the session to explain the benefits of direct communication with LEP patients.

5. **They hold you responsible for the patient's actions.**
"But remember last time you were here, she agreed to take her pills?" "But he needed to come this morning NPO!" "Can't you get her to stop ________ (*insert any undesirable behavior here*)?" Again, as the calm professional, you can either interpret the question, tell the provider you don't know but would be happy to interpret, or gently remind the provider of your role. Sometimes these sorts of outbursts are simply rhetorical questions representing the provider's frustration with patient non-compliance; he or she doesn't really expect an answer. It is still important for you not to get drawn into this dynamic.

6. **They say things, which they then ask you not to interpret.**
Even when you do a pre-session, some providers seem unable to contain their side comments. Personally, I use the "two-strikes-you're-out" rule. The first time a provider does this, I do not interpret but gently remind him or her that I am obligated to interpret everything that is said. That puts the provider on notice. If it happens again, I interpret the comment. Providers rapidly learn to use me as an interpreter, not a confidant.

7. **They ask you to consent the patient.**
Perhaps we should be flattered when providers leave us alone with the consent form and ask us to "go over" it with the patient. After all, they are putting their patient's understanding and their own professional license in our hands. Still, interpreters cannot be answering questions about procedures, risks, alternative treatments, etc.; we are not physicians. Consenting a patient is both an ethical and a legal process, and we must insist that providers stay present to get consent and to answer questions.

8. **They correct your interpretation.**
Now, I ask myself, do I correct the provider's diagnosis? Or critique her surgical technique? Or take exception to his interpretation of an echocardiogram? Of course not! But, again, many providers are unaware of the role of the interpreter or the difficulty of interpreting

meaning accurately. They may be accustomed to working with unqualified interpreters whose work they have good reason to question. It is important, then, that we not get defensive when this happens, but simply respond to the content of the correction; no, the interpretation was accurate, or yes, the patient's words could be interpreted another way. Calm is the key; leave the ego outside the room. A word to the provider after the session, however, might be appropriate.

9. **They complain to your agency about behavior that was entirely ethical and within the National Standards of Practice.**
   This is my favorite! There is nothing more frustrating than having a complaint sent in about behavior that was completely appropriate for a professional interpreter. The good news is that a good agency carefully investigates each complaint and is not shy about using the opportunity to educate clients and providers if need be. Do what you know to be good practice, and your agency should back you up.

Conclusion

Wouldn't it be nice, though, if providers would just stop doing these things? In fact, educational programs in medical schools, residency programs and continuing education programs are helping current and future generations of healthcare professionals better understand the role and practice of professional interpreters, leading to fewer "difficult docs" and better teamwork between providers and interpreters on the healthcare team.

September, 2006

29.

Why Don't They Just Learn English?

(Author's note: Many of the facts cited in this article come from *Hold Your Tongue: Bilingualism and the Politics of "English Only"* by James Crawford, published by Addison-Wesley Publishing Company. I highly recommend it.)

Have you ever tried to explain to your family, friends, and casual acquaintances exactly what you do? Here's a typical exchange for me.

New acquaintance: "So, what do you do for a living?"

Me: "I work in Language Access in Health Care."

New acquaintance: "Excuse me?"

Me: "I train medical interpreters."

New acquaintance: "What?"

Me: "Medical interpreters."

New acquaintance: "You mean, like those folks who type up the notes the doctor records about patients?"

Me: "No, not quite. When a patient who doesn't speak English comes to the hospital, and if the doctor doesn't speak the patient's language, I interpret so that they can both understand each other."

New acquaintance: "Oh, like at the United Nations, right? Gee, that's interesting. (*pause*) Could I get one of you guys to go in with me? I can't understand a word my doctor says!"

Most of the time, people I meet think my work is really interesting. Sometimes, however, I get a different response. Sometimes, the person I'm talking with doesn't think my chosen profession is so useful. Instead, I may be asked why scarce resources are being spent on more services for "them." Eventually, the question comes up: "Why don't they just learn English?"

"After all," they say, "English is the official language of the United States and always has been. If immigrants and refugees come here, they should learn English and not expect the taxpayers here to pay for them to have interpreters. As it is, immigrants already get a free ride in this country, what with education and health care. When everyone else's grandparents and great grandparents came to the U.S., nobody helped them, and they all learned English right away. Immigrants these days don't even try to learn English. Interpreter services are a waste of money that could be better spent on benefiting more of us."

Well, that's what I hear, anyway. But surprisingly, when you look at the facts, a lot of these commonly accepted statements are not quite so black and white. Let's take a look at these common myths about language in the United States.

"English is, and always has been, the official language of the United States."

Actually, believe it or not, English is not the official language of the United States. The U.S. has no official language. The framers of the Constitution considered specifying a national language for their fledgling nation, and chose not to, based on the great linguistic diversity found in the country.

Certainly, English is the lingua franca in this country: the language of business, education and politics. And I, at least, am not suggesting that new arrivals to this country should not learn English; there is a very limited future in store for those who do not learn the language of the land.

However, if you remember your high-school history, you'll remember that the U.S. has always been a country of different cultural and linguistic groups. Before European contact, Native American nations spoke between 500 and 1000 different languages. In 1664, New York City was home to significant populations speaking 18 different languages, including English, Dutch, German, Swedish and French. Few of us know that the Continental Congress translated many of its documents into German and French as a means of building public support. The Louisiana Purchase in 1803 added a huge monolingual French-speaking community to the country, and the legal and political systems of Louisiana functioned bilingually for almost a century after that. Minnesota's constitution was published in 1857 in five languages. And when the most of the Southwest was transferred from Mexican to U.S. ownership in 1848, the Treaty of Guadalupe Hidalgo guaranteed the rights of the residents to run their personal and civic affairs in Spanish. And in more modern times, the 2000 census tells us that nearly 47 million people - 18 percent of the U.S. population - speak a language other than English at home. Immigrants and refugees do need to learn English. However, to paint the American nation as a monolithic English-speaking country is to ignore the truth of our historic and valuable diversity.

"Immigrants and refugees come here for a free ride and expect too many services in return."

Refugees come to the United States running for their lives. Most would much rather have stayed home, thank you very much, except that home had become too dangerous. The truth of refugee resettlement is that most refugees don't get a choice as to where they are going; they are sent to the first country that will take them.

Immigrants do choose to come; some more than others. Most come for economic reasons, because there is no work in their country of origin, and because they want to find a better life for their families. And, statistically speaking, new immigrants are some of the hardest working people in the country. It is not unusual in immigrant communities for people to be working two or three jobs: most often the lowest-paying, dirtiest and most taxing jobs in agriculture, in meat packing, in the food and textile industries. Without immigrant labor, the cost of the food we eat would skyrocket. In addition, immigrants pay taxes like everyone else and contribute to the economy by spending their income. While immigrants do benefit from the educational system in the U.S, changes in federal policies have severely restricted the other sorts of social benefits that immigrants can count on in many states, such as access to Medicaid, Medicare, SSI or unemployment.

As a matter of fact, a recent study in the State of Virginia looked at the net input of immigrants to the state economy compared to the net cost of publicly funded benefits. The researchers came to the conclusion that the immigrants were a net economic benefit to the state. So much for the "free ride" theory.

"My grandparents came as immigrants and nobody ever helped them. They learned English. Immigrants and refugees today aren't learning English fast enough. Most of them never even try to learn."

Most of us either are immigrants or the descendants of immigrants. And almost all immigrant groups follow the same pattern, regardless of whether they came in 1892 or

1992: they band together with others who share their language and culture for mutual help and emotional comfort. Today's immigrants are no more isolated and intent on maintaining their language of origin than those of a century ago. As a matter of fact, more recent waves of immigrants are learning English and acculturating faster than any previous wave in U.S. history. However, we do not often provide the support they need. The day in 1986 that Californians voted to make English the official language of the state, there were over 40,000 people on waiting lists for ESL classes in Los Angeles alone. This is not the portrait of a group of people refusing to learn English.

"Language access services are for the benefit of the patient."

We often talk about interpreter services being for the patient. This is largely because the early advances in providing interpreters in health care came out of Civil Rights complaints and legal litigation. But think about it for a moment. Healthcare providers need interpreters just as much as the patients do. Research is showing us that not having interpreters leads to more expensive health care in the end, and that the cost is paid by all of us through insurance premiums. And from a public health point of view, none of us benefit when a person with active tuberculosis, or hepatitis, or HIV, or SARS is left untreated to infect others in the community. We all pay when a whole sector of the society can't get access to good health care. Looking at it that way, language access services benefit us all.

Conclusion

There are some folks in the U.S. who are just xenophobic – meaning, they are frightened of anyone who is different than they. But many Americans simply need to be educated. It's not a case of "us" and "them." "They" **are** "us." All of us are "we." English is still the *lingua franca* of the U.S. and immigrants are learning to speak it. But the ER and the cancer ward are not the right places to be practicing, not when the potential consequences of miscommunication are so profound. In the end, we all benefit from being a multilingual society, and we all benefit from clear communication in health care.

So, come to think of it, until doctors learn to speak plain English, sending in interpreters with all patients might not be such a bad idea either . . .

April 2004

Section 4

R_X for Interpreters

30.

Staying Healthy While Serving the Sick

Have you ever thought that you have a potentially dangerous job? I'm not referring to rocketing through traffic to make it to your next assignment on time, or getting stuck in the elevator on the 11th floor of the medical center, or dodging the Doberman who's guarding the door at your 3:00 home visit. I'm talking about all the nasty little germs that float around medical centers where sick people go for care. Yuck! They got sick from those things – how do you avoid getting sick too?

At this point, all you telephonic interpreters out there are saying, "Wow, I'm glad I work over the telephone!" In fact, one of the indications for using telephonic interpreting is when the patient is either highly infectious, or when the patient's immune system is so compromised that exposure to germs from the interpreter could jeopardize the patient's health. But for the many on-site interpreters who are reading this, the advice in today's article is extremely important. So pay attention! (And all you telephonic interpreters can take a break . . .)

Like everyone else who works in health care, on-site interpreters need to learn and follow a set of procedures knows as "Universal Precautions." Sounds like a way to save the galaxy, doesn't it? Well, whatever it sounds like, these procedures can help you stay healthy while being surrounded by folks who are sick. The whole point of taking Universal Precautions is to prevent you from coming in contact with any potentially infectious material - blood, sputum, urine, air-borne contaminants, etc. Since we don't know when somebody's body fluids may be infected, some precautions we take all the time. In cases where we know a patient is infected, we sometimes take extra precautions.

Precautions we should take all the time:

Hand washing

Yes, I know, I sound like your Mom, but you know, she was right. Washing your hands after every patient encounter is one of the most effective ways to stop infection. As a medical interpreter, your physical contact with patients is usually limited to shaking hands at most, and you should never be handling instruments, supplies or specimens. Regardless, it is a good idea to wash your hands between appointments. Wash your hands with soap, lathering up for at least 15 seconds. Rinse thoroughly, dry your hands with a paper towel, and turn the faucets off with those towels.

Vaccinations

Many health care workers like to keep their vaccinations up to date, and an increasing number of hospitals are requiring these vaccinations of all their staff and contractors. Vaccinations for Hepatitis B and for Influenza are often recommended for people who have direct patient contact. Consult with your primary care physician about whether such immunizations would be right for you.

Other precautions we take only under certain circumstances:

Personal Protective Equipment

PPE is specialized clothing or equipment that protects you against exposure to infectious materials. Masks, gowns, gloves and protective eyewear are all examples of PPE. Again, as a medical interpreter, you will rarely be required to wear a mask or gown, but if you are interpreting in an operating room or in an isolation ward, or if you are interpreting for a patient with active TB, you may need to use PPE. Take your cue from the providers; if they are masked, you should be masked too. Also, keep an eye out for signs that specify use of PPE and ask hospital staff if you have any questions.

In radiology

Whenever X-rays are in use, you should either stand behind the lead shield like the radiologist and the radiology technician, or you should be wearing a lead apron and gorget (throat shield). If you suspect you may be pregnant, you should not accept appointments in which X-ray technology is used: this includes simple X-rays, barium enemas, barium swallows (upper GI series), hysterosalpingograms, CT scans and others.

In mental health settings

If you are interpreting in a mental health setting, ask the provider before starting as to the patient's state of mind. If the patient is psychotic or has a tendency for violence, adjust your positioning to maintain some distance between yourself and the patient.

A few other issues

What to do if you think you may have been exposed to infection? If for some reason, you have sustained an injury in the hospital and you think you may have been exposed to infectious material, immediately clean the injury with soap and running water. Notify staff immediately and fill out a written accident report within one day. Consult with your physician as to whether you need any sort of medical treatment or prophylaxis.

If you've been interpreting for a patient who is later found to have active tuberculosis, get a TB test done immediately in order to establish if you have been exposed to TB previously. Then, about three months later, get another test. This second test will tell if you have been infected by the patient and whether you need treatment.

There is one other area to consider in keeping yourself well, and this is where you telephonic interpreters need to start paying attention again. Healthcare interpreting can expose you not only to potential physical infection, it can wear you down emotionally. I have dealt in other articles with taking care of your mental health as an interpreter; you might want to go back and read those. Maintaining professional boundaries, finding someone to talk to (while maintaining confidentiality, of course), eating right, taking breaks, and finding a personally satisfying way to blow off steam are all important "universal precautions" to help protect you from emotional burn-out. Unfortunately, there's no PPE to protect you from the pain of a dying child nor a vaccine to immunize you against sympathizing with the patients you serve. These things are part of the work we do. But the more physical and emotional hand-washing we do, the more we can keep ourselves physically and psychologically healthy, and the more likely it is that we'll be available to help all the patients who need us.

August, 2005

31.

Taking Care of Business

Tips for the Independent Contractor

When someone asks you what you do for a living, I'll bet you answer, "I'm an interpreter." Have you ever thought of answering, "I own my own business"?

Most of us don't think of ourselves as small business owners. We rarely come to interpreting with an MBA, but rather with a love of language and a desire to be of service to the community. As a result, most of us have no idea about what setting up a business entails. So, in the spirit of supporting professional development, this article is written to give interpreters who are independent contractors some suggestions on how to set up and manage their interpreting business.

Step 1: Choose professionals to help you.

You will definitely benefit from having an accountant (a CPA), if only to help with your taxes. It is also a good idea to make friends with your banker when you open your business account. As your business grows, you may also want to have a lawyer and an insurance agent who can help you get liability insurance.

Step 2: Decide whether to be a sole proprietorship or an LLC.

A sole proprietorship is set up such that the owner essentially is the company. A Limited Liability Corporation (LLC) is an entity on its own, from which the owner takes the profits. The important difference for business owners is that if someone wins a suit against a sole proprietorship, they can get all the owner's assets, both business and personal. A winning suit against an LLC gives the winner access only to the company's assets, not the owner's assets. It takes just a little more effort to set up as an LLC, however that little bit of effort could protect you later on.

Step 3: Get a business license, if required.

In many states and cities you need to have a business license in order to run your own business, if you earn over a certain amount of money. Such a Master Business License will come with a Unified Business Identifier number (UBI). Usually the registration fees are quite small. So check with your state and city Department of Licensing to find out what is required in order to establish your business legally.

Step 4: Get an EIN number.

It's a very good idea to get a federal Employee Identification Number from the Internal Revenue Service (IRS). This is the number you can give companies that want to contract for your services, instead of your Social Security number. Due to problems with identity theft, it is a good idea not to have your Social Security number in the hands of too many people. To get an EIN, you need to fill out an SS-4 form. Or you can apply for and receive your EIN electronically from the IRS website at www.irs.gov/businesses/small/article/0,,id=102767,00.html.

Step 5: Open a business bank account.

One of the most common errors we small business owners make is co-mingling our personal and business finances. While it sure seems a lot easier in the short run to just deposit checks into and pay business expenses out of our personal accounts, this makes record-keeping much more difficult and, if we ever get audited, makes the IRS folks very grumpy. And believe me, you don't want to make the IRS auditor grumpy.

So go to your bank and set up a business account. This is the account your checks go into, this is the account from which you pay your business expenses, and this is the account from which you transfer money into your personal account for your personal use. A little extra effort, but it keeps the boundaries very clear.

Step 6: Set up an accounting program.

It is important to keep financial records of your business, both for you and for the IRS. There are a number of commercial products out there that are designed just for small business owners like us. Here are a few:

- Intuit QuickBooks or Quicken

- Microsoft Money Home and Business
- Ledger / Shoebox Accounting

Find one you like and learn to use it. It may seem a headache at first, but once you get adept at using the program, it will be easy.

Now you're set up and ready to go. A business, however, also requires care and feeding to keep it healthy. As you go along:

Keep records.

It is important to develop a system to record your income (accounts receivable) and your expenses (accounts payable) on an on-going basis. Personally, I stick all my receipts and check stubs in a folder, and I designate one day at the end of each month to enter everything into QuickBooks. If you have many receipts, you might want to do this weekly. The key is to find a schedule that works for you and stick to it. You really don't want to get to December 31 and have to input everything for the whole year all at once. Trust me on this one. Really.

Pay your taxes.

You all know that you must pay federal income taxes on what you earn. As a small business owner, you can still file a 1040 form, but you must also fill out a Schedule C (Profit or Loss from Business). If you work from a home office and you want to take a deduction for that, you must also fill out Form 8829. A good accountant can help you with this.

Taxes aren't something to worry about only in April, however. If you worked as an employee, your employer would pay your SSI and withhold money from every paycheck toward your federal taxes. As an independent business owner you will need to do both for yourself. The former you will pay through self-employment taxes as part of your federal tax return. The latter you will need to pay to the IRS quarterly, on April 15, June 15, September 15 and January 15. Late or underpayment of your quarterly taxes can cost you in fines.[15]

Depending on where you live, you may also have to pay state and city business taxes, and perhaps city business taxes. Check with your state and city Departments of Revenue to make sure you're clear on your responsibilities.

As a small business owner, it can feel as if you are charged a great deal in taxes. However, businesses can also take many deductions, **if you keep receipts and records**

---

[15] So, from every check, put 30% into a separate account so you will always have money to pay your taxes.

of them. These include:

- Mileage: any driving you do for business purposes, even if it is to the store to buy office supplies, can be noted down. At the end of the year, you can multiple your miles by the federal mileage reimbursement rate and take that as an expense. You can find the government's current rates at www.gsa.gov.

- Parking: any parking expenses related to business can be taken as expenses.

- Professional dues or membership: the membership fees for joining the National Council on Interpreting in Health Care, CHIA or any other professional interpreting association can be taken as an expense.

- Professional subscriptions: do you subscribe to any interpreting magazines? The subscription cost can be taken as well.

- Licensure or testing fees: the cost of getting certified or getting those licenses mentioned above can be taken as expenses.

- Travel/lodging/food expenses when traveling on business

- Postage/mailing

- Office supplies

- Photocopying

- Advertising and printing, such as business cards

- Capital equipment expense, such as a computer, a printer, a headset, office furniture.

- Home office deductions: if you work from a home office, calculate the percent of your home's total square footage that is represented by your home office. Then you can deduct this percentage of your total utility costs as well - that means electricity, water, sewer, garbage/ recycling, etc.

- Health insurance premiums and out of pocket medical costs

- Communication costs: Pager, cell phone, telephone, long distance charges
- City and state business taxes

Conclusion

"What a hassle!" You're thinking. Being your own boss does require some organization and consistent effort. On the other hand, it provides you with a certain independence that being an employee does not. And once you get your business set up, and your maintenance systems in place, you can return your attention to the real reason you're in business for yourself – your love of interpreting.

February, 2007

32.

Interpreting in Small Communities

Keeping Both your Job and your Friends

I'm going to write this month about something with which I have no experience at all. Yet I have heard from many interpreters who struggle with this problem, and who have come up with interesting strategies to address it. The challenge: living and interpreting in a small community.

A "small community" can be defined geographically (such as a small town) or demographically (such as a small language community). Whether you're interpreting in Ukiah, OR (population 256) or in the Somali community in Los Angeles, you probably face the same issues. You know almost everybody you interpret for, and they know you. Professional distance is a myth when everyone knows your phone number and you see your patients at church (or the temple or the mosque) on Sunday (or Friday). People expect more from you because you are not just "the interpreter:" you are their neighbor, their friend, their link to the wider society. You owe them a loyalty, because of the community you share, and this makes your job even harder than usual.

This problem manifests itself in a variety of ways. Patients may call you at home, asking for your help interpreting (for free, of course) in venues where you haven't been contracted. They may ask you to fill out forms for them or to help them call the electric company to figure out a bill. They may ask you about other patients whom you know in common, often out of sincere concern for the patient's well being. They may ask you how to get what they need from the hospital; they may ask you to lie for them; they may want you to use your influence to fix a problem; they may need a ride to their appointment; they may want your advice on their medical problems. And, at least at first, you may very well want to help them, because helping people is one reason you went into medical interpreting. But some of the things your patients will want are violations of the Code of Ethics. Some will be against hospital rules. And some will simply eat you alive as more and more patients make more and more demands on your time.

What can you do then, as an interpreter in a small community, to keep both your job and your friends? How do you -- as Margaret Lavallee, a Cree interpreter from Manitoba, asked -- maintain credibility with both your home community and your professional community? A lot of it has to do with deciding how much you **want** to do, what you are **willing** to do, and with **managing expectations**. Here are some of the strategies that interpreters have told me they use.

1. Establish very clear boundaries with your patients, in and out of the hospital.

This is the "I'm sorry, I don't work on Sundays" option. It means helping patients be clear about what they can and cannot expect of you. This means you have to be clear with yourself about what you are willing to do and what you will not do. Of course, patients may become angry with you when they want more than you can give. They may accuse you of forgetting where you come from or of abandoning your own folk. They may gossip about you in the community. If you choose this option, you'll just have to be pleasant and polite and firm - and live with whatever frustration your patients express.

2. Accept a role as community language liaison.

This is the "It's OK, I'm always up at 2:00 a.m." option. In this option, you choose to widen your boundaries enough to live up to everyone's expectations. This will work fine until you burn out or you find yourself in a position in which the patient's expectations and the institution's expectations of you are diametrically opposed. Then you'll have to choose to either help the patient and potentially lose your job or do what your employer expects and potentially lose your friend.

3. Sidestep

Notice I didn't say "lie," exactly. In some communities it is considered exceptionally rude to say "no," but there are lots of ways of saying "yes" that convey the same meaning. Yes, I'd love to help you fill out that form, but I don't have any time at all until next week. Of course, I'd love to give you a ride, but I'm going to be at the hospital already for an earlier appointment. How's Mrs. Gutierrez doing? You know,

I don't really know. What to do about your back problem? Wow, that's a hard one; I'd ask your doctor, if I were you. If this sort of indirect communication is a cultural norm in your community, you may find this is a softer way of helping patients understand your limitations. If you come from a culture that values more direct styles of communication, this approach may be seen as being devious, disrespectful and dishonest. You'll have to decide.

4. Ask your employer to set limits.

This is the "I can't - I'll get fired!" option. In this option, you control expectations by having someone else (your boss) create the boundary, so that you won't be held responsible for it. This is often an effective strategy for limiting expectations of you at work, but it doesn't do much to limit community expectations of you outside of work.

5. Find another way to provide interpreter services.

I jokingly call this the "Run away!" option. It means moving yourself into a work situation in which you can meet everybody's expectations. You may choose to only interpret in the next town over or move to a bigger city. Interpreters in small ethnic communities may choose to work through a telephonic interpreting service, so that most of their clients are on the other side of the country. While this is certainly a loss for the community, each interpreter has the right to find a work situation in which he or she can be productive and happy.

A final challenge related to interpreting in small communities is interpreting for people you know and having too much information about them. Our professional Code of Ethics prohibits us from interpreting for close friends and family, since it is almost impossible to be impartial in these cases. But in small communities, you may know just about everyone well. This means that you'll have to be extremely careful to respect confidentiality in the community; if you slip, your reputation as a "talker" will assure that nobody will want you as an interpreter. You may also find that you know when patients are lying or telling only part of the truth. Just remember that it is not your responsibility to share information about the patient that you know from your associations in the community, nor is it your responsibility to point out lies. You may know that the patient drinks; you are under no obligation to tell the doctor. You may know that your patient does not qualify for the hospital discount; the lie is the patient's, not yours. Sometimes knowing too much about your patient is a real burden, but it is part and parcel of living in a small community.

Conclusion

There is, of course, a bright side to interpreting in small communities. There are few joys greater than being of service to people of whom you feel you are a part. There are few satisfactions as great as receiving the respect and trust of your own community. And, though sometimes the object of frustration and anger, a community's interpreter is a vital link to the wider society, to the services and opportunities this country has to offer. If you can find that balance between what you want to give, what you can give and what the community expects of you, you have a real chance to be that vital link. And still keep your friends.

November, 2005

33.

For the Public Good

Volunteering Your Services

For years I have been urging you interpreters to get trained, to continue your education, to deepen your ethical awareness, to hone your skills, and to practice, practice, practice until you become exceptional in your chosen field. I've encouraged you to be true professionals and to demand to be treated as professionals.

Today I am going to urge you to give it all away. For free.

Don't panic; I'm not suggesting that you rip up your next invoice to Pacific Interpreters. All of us need to earn a living, and interpreters should be paid a respectable wage in return for their substantial skills. I am suggesting that you join many other professionals in offering a small portion of your time and professional expertise pro bono to organizations that cannot pay for them. Call it a little payback to the country that has given us so much.

The term "pro bono" comes from the Latin term *pro bono publico*, which means "for the public good." Working pro bono, or volunteering, is an important aspect of being a professional and of being a member of a community. It helps create the kind of society in which we all want to live. It allows us to help others in need of assistance. And it provides an important role model for our children, demonstrating the importance that service to others holds in our lives.

On June 23, 1975, author Erma Bombeck published a commentary on volunteering in her nationally syndicated column. It so impressed me that I cut it out and saved it. I reproduce it here, in part.

> *I had a dream the other night that every volunteer in this country, disillusioned with the lack of compassion, had set sail for another country . . .*
>
> *As I stood smiling on the pier, I shouted "Good-bye phone committees. So long Disease of the Month . . . Au revoir playground duty, bake sales and three-hour meetings.*
>
> *As the boat got smaller and they could no longer hear my shouts, I reflected, serves them right. A bunch of yes people . . . Oh well, who needs them!*
>
> *The hospital was quiet as I passed it. Rooms were void of books, flowers and voices. The children's wing held no clowns . . . no laughter. The reception desk was vacant.*
>
> *The Home for the Aged was like a tomb. The blind listened for a voice that never came. The infirm were imprisoned by wheels on a chair that never moved. Food grew cold on trays that would never reach the mouths of the hungry.*
>
> *All the social agencies had closed their doors, unable to implement their programs of scouting, recreation, drug control, Big Sisters, Big Brothers, YW, YM, the retarded, the crippled, the lonely, and the abandoned . . .*
>
> *The schools were strangely quiet with no field trips, no volunteer aids on the playground or in the classrooms . . . as were the colleges where scholarships and financial support were no more.*
>
> *The flowers on church altars withered and died. Children in day nurseries lifted their arms, but there was no one to hold them in love. Alcoholics cried out in despair, but no one answered and the poor had no recourse for health care or legal aid . . .*
>
> *I fought in my sleep to regain a glimpse of the ship of volunteers just one more time. It was to be my last glimpse of civilization . . . as we were meant to be.*

Of course, it is worthwhile to volunteer your time in any way that has meaning to you. However, as interpreters, you have very specific and vitally needed skills that will be welcomed by many organizations. While institutions that receive federal funding are required to provide interpreters, there are many small community agencies whose funding is private and limited and who cannot afford to pay for professional interpreters. Nevertheless, their services are vital to non-English speakers who are struggling here in the U.S. Volunteering for even a few hours a week can provide a vital service to them and a unique satisfaction for you.

Here are a few organizations that will most likely welcome your language skills, your interpreting skills or both.

- **The American Red Cross (ARC)** is desperately seeking both bilingual caseworkers and interpreters. During the response to Hurricane Katrina, it became clear that the Red Cross needed more volunteers who spoke languages other than English, as well as interpreters, to assist the victims of the disaster. Imagine the agony of losing everything in a hurricane and then not being able to get help because you don't speak English! Even if you cannot travel to the site of large regional disasters like Katrina, the Red Cross also needs your help in responding to local tragedies such as apartment fires, floods, etc. Contact your local chapter of the Red Cross to see how you can best serve. Some chapters, like those in Boston and Seattle, have well organized volunteer Language Banks to provide interpreters to Emergency Response Teams and community organizations. If your local chapter doesn't have one, help organize one!

[Author's update: If you are interested in interpreting for the Red Cross during major national or international disasters, the National Association of Judicial Interpreters and Translators (NAJIT) has signed a memorandum of understanding with ARC to recruit and screen interpreters who are needed for specific work in affected areas. For example, after the disastrous 2010 earthquake in Haiti, NAJIT helped recruit volunteer translators and medical interpreters to serve month-long stints on the hospital ship USNS Comfort. You can contact NAJIT at www.najit.org.]

- Unlike most health care and social service agencies, **homeless shelters and domestic violence shelters** are often run on donations alone, with neither a federal mandate nor the budget to provide professional interpretation. Still, these agencies serve large numbers of non-English-speaking clients with a serious need for help. Women's shelters in particular need highly skilled interpreters who can handle both the emotional trauma and the legal challenges that face victims of domestic violence.

- **Food banks** can either be a lifesaver or a confusing source of frustration for clients who don't speak English. Again, most food banks operate on extremely limited private funding and cannot justify hiring professional interpreters. However food banks serving communities with many limited-English-proficient families will be very grateful to have access to volunteers who can help both to bridge the language gap and to make the food bank offerings a better match to the diet of culturally diverse populations.

- **Legal Aid programs,** especially those working on issues of immigrant rights, serve large numbers of LEP clients. Many of the lawyers working for these groups are providing their services pro bono and would welcome the support of professional interpreters. These services cover client-lawyer communications only, not formal court proceedings, but knowledge of legal terminology will certainly help.

- **HIV/AIDS** community outreach and counseling programs need bilingual outreach workers as well as interpreters. Those of you who do medical interpreting are uniquely qualified to assist these groups.

Conclusion

There will be other community service groups where you live that could benefit from your volunteer help. Find one that matches your passion, and, *pro bono publico*, use your skills to make your community a better place.

January, 2006

34.

Attend a Convention, Get Energized!

Conference season is coming up and there is no better time than now to start planning which one(s) you are going to attend!

What is this resounding silence I am hearing? You aren't planning on going to any conferences this year? They're too expensive? They're boring? They're scary? You won't learn anything because you know it all already???

Well, phooey on you. You need to rethink! Conferences are an important way to keep in touch with your field, improve your skills, and meet people who, like yourself, actually know the difference between a translator and an interpreter. Let's see if we can address some of those excuses.

"Conferences are too expensive."

Well, expensive is, of course, a relative term, and conferences do cost money for registration, travel, lodging and food. Here are some ways to make conference-going less expensive:

- To reduce registration costs, choose a conference that fits your budget. Join the association that is running the conference so as to qualify for a member discount. And register early to get the lower "early bird" rates.

- To reduce travel costs, pick a conference close to home. Or, pick one that is taking place in a "hub" city, to which you can fly for a relatively cheap rate. Use frequent flyer miles, and buy your ticket early.

- To reduce lodging costs, share a hotel room with a friend who is also attending. Most hotels will let you put up to four people in a room for the same price as one. Make sure you book your room early so you get one of the limited number of discounted rooms negotiated by the conference organizers. Another strategy is to stay at a cheaper hotel close to the conference hotel.

- Some conferences offer scholarships. Check with the organizers; maybe you will qualify.

- If you are an independent businessperson (contract or freelance interpreter), remember to take the expenses related to conference attendance as a deduction on your federal income tax!

"Conferences are boring and/or scary."

Conferences, like wild animals, can be boring or scary if you don't know how to approach them. If you're going for the first time, make a point of sitting down with the program when you get there, reading the abstracts and choosing the sessions you want to attend. Mark them with a highlighter to make the program easier to follow. Ask around about who the good presenters are; sometimes it's worth going to a presentation in which you're only moderately interested if the presenter is particularly skilled.

There are also a lot of ancillary activities at conferences that make them more fun:

- Pre-conference sessions – longer workshops focused on skill development – are typically offered by nationally known trainers and represent a great learning opportunity.

- Exhibitors will be happy to show you their wares, describe their services, sign you up for things and give you neat little gadgets with their logos on them.

- Evening activities may include dinner dances, film festivals, social outings, etc.

"What could I possibly learn?"

Do I really have to answer this one? No matter how good we are as interpreters, we can always learn something more: vocabulary, interpreting skills, a new way of looking at our role, trends in the field, new technologies. Most importantly, going to a conference will put you smack in the middle of a large group of people who share your passion for interpreting. Finally! Someone with whom to swap stories, someone from whom to ask advice; someone who understands.

And that right there may be worth the whole price of admission.

February 2009

35.

A Healthcare Interpreter's Guide to Testing—Part I

Some of you may remember the days when all you needed to do to become an interpreter was to say you spoke a language other than English. Thank goodness, those days are (mostly) gone! As healthcare interpreting develops from an ad-hoc activity to a recognized profession, the requirements to become an interpreter are becoming more stringent. And chances are that you have been, or soon will be, tested to prove that you really do have the knowledge, skills and attitudes necessary to serve as a competent interpreter. As a matter of fact, one way or another, national certification is on its way, and you can bet that it will include a test.

OK, I see about a third of you out there cheering, a third of you are looking decidedly grumpy, and a third of you look like you may run screaming from the room. To the second group, I say, "Cheer up! Testing is not so bad!" To the third group, I say, "Don't panic! You can do this." And to the first group I say, "Wow, that's really weird - who likes being tested?"

Very few of us really enjoy taking tests. But those folks in celebratory Group Number One recognize that a fair, transparent, valid and reliable testing process is important both to assure that interpreters really are competent and to build confidence in our skills among those who depend on them - patients and providers.

Whether you welcome testing, resent being tested or faint at the thought of taking a test, this article will help you understand more about testing and how to prepare for an interpreter skills assessment.

Three things you should know about tests

There are a lot of assessment tools being used in the healthcare interpreting world today. As interpreters, we aren't generally given the choice of which test we'd like to take. However, there are some things you should know about assessments that will help you be more aware of issues regarding testing.

1. **Not all tests are created equal.**
   In the world of psychometrics (the field that includes testing), there are tests, and then there are Tests. Anyone can sit down in an office, write up ten multiple-choice questions and have a test. And for some purposes, that is just fine. Teachers, for example, write tests based on what they have taught to see how much their students have retained and what the class may need to go over again. But for "high stakes tests" - those are tests that determine whether someone can work or how much they will earn - you want to use a testing instrument that has been scientifically developed and that is valid and reliable.

   What does it mean that a test is valid and reliable? Validity means that the test actually measures what it says it measures. We look for validity in content and in construct. The test's content, for example, should reflect knowledge related to the tested topic. So, we don't require students to analyze a poem on a biology test, and we shouldn't ask interpreters to diagnose disease from a case study on an interpreting test. Construct validity means that taking the test does not require skills other than the ones being tested. So, a test of language skills should not require the candidate to interpret - that's a different skill. A test of oral language ability should not require reading and writing - those are different skills too.

   The most valid test for an interpreter, then, would be for raters to observe an interpreter during an actual interpreting encounter. Of course, this is not possible in most cases, so we have to compromise somewhat on construct validity. A test of interpreting skills will probably require some skills not technically required of an interpreter: for example, reading, writing or perhaps using a computer to take the test. A good test of interpreting skills, however, will minimize the use of non-essential skills and provide alternative methods of testing for candidates who feel that those non-essential testing methods are actually creating a barrier to them demonstrating the essential skills. So validity is actually testing what you say you are testing, and only that. Reliability, on the other hand, means that a given candidate will get the same score regardless of which form of a test he takes, who administers it, when he takes it, who rates it, when it is rated and if it is re-rated later. Reliability depends on careful selection, training, and supervision of test administrators and test raters. Administrators must be trained to give the test the same way to all candidates. Raters must be trained to rate consistently so that they all rate a given candidate's test the same. The degree to which raters' scoring agrees with each other is called inter-rater reliability. An inter-rater reliability of 1.0 (which is highly unusual) means that all the raters came up with the exact same score on a candidate's test. Scores of .9 or .8 are still good. Below that, you may start to wonder whether your failing grade was due to your performance or to the person who graded your test.

2. **Not all testing organizations are equally credible.**
   A test's credibility depends a great deal on how it was developed, who is implementing it and what conflicts of interest come into play. For example, let's say an interpreting test is offered not-for-profit by a university. The university has no stake in whether a given candidate passes the test or not; it doesn't gain anything by failing candidates or passing them. There is no conflict of interest. On the other hand, consider a large telephonic interpreting company offering to test the interpreters at a hospital where it provides telephonic interpreting. The fewer interpreters pass the company's test, the more the hospital has to use the company's telephonic interpreters. The company has a vested interest in failing the hospital's interpreters, so there is a conflict of interest. Whether or not the company actually does fail candidates in order to boost its own business is irrelevant; the fact that it has a vested interest to do so creates the conflict and makes that company an inappropriate testing organization for that hospital. Where there is trust, one can sometimes work around conflicts of interest. So if you see a conflict of interest, you must ask yourself, "Do I trust this entity to test my skills fairly?"

3. **Valid and reliable tests are costly to develop, implement and maintain.**
   Though one might imagine that the result of a test development

process is a single test, that is not the case. In high-stakes testing, test developers write, test and adapt enough test items to have a pool of about ten items for every one on the test. So if a test has five questions related to confidentiality, the developers really have a pool of 50 questions on confidentiality. Different forms of the test will have different but equivalent questions. New items are constantly under development and old items are retired. As a result, early candidates can't tell later candidates what questions will be on the test, and those who retake the test will get an equivalent test with different questions.

All of this is part of test development and, of course, costs money. Implementing a high-stakes test is also expensive. Testing organizations have to pay for test administrators and test raters, communication with candidates and marketing. Depending on how the test is administered, the testing organization may also have to pay for space, scheduling, computer software and testing equipment. If the testing organization is a commercial entity, it will also want to take a profit.

In addition, high-stakes tests need to be maintained over time. For example, even raters who have excellent inter-rater reliability tend to drift off the standard; their work needs to be periodically checked and retraining done, usually on an annual basis. New items need to be continually developed, tested and integrated into test forms. Security breaches need to be handled. And, of course, new test administrators and raters will need to be recruited and trained to replace raters who move on to other work.

In short, it takes money to develop and maintain a testing program. Depending on the testing organization, grant funding may play a part in underwriting the initial development. Maintenance, however, will always require income from test fees. So, if you are asked to undergo testing to work as an interpreter, be prepared to pay for it. Remember though, through the pain of writing that check, that this is a valuable investment in your professional future, a proof of your competence as an interpreter. Plus, if you're an independent contractor, you can always take it off your income tax!

Summary so far . . .

Healthcare interpreting is moving slowly out of the realm of low-stakes, informal testing into the world of high-stakes standardized testing: tests that should be valid and reliable and that likely will be costly. But this shift should not be a source of worry for working interpreters. Instead, we need to learn how to successfully prepare for and take these tests. In my next article, I'll share some ideas about what tends to be on interpreter skills tests and how to prepare for such a test, as well as some little secrets about taking standardized tests. Because whether or not you join Group Number One in cheering the thought of more testing, assessment is coming, and with some preparation you can handle it.

April 2009

36.

A Healthcare Interpreter's Guide to Testing – Part II

Or The Top Twelve Tips for Test Taking

In Part I of this series, I wrote about the impending reality of interpreter skills testing. Yes, like it or not, you will most probably be asked in the next several years to prove your interpreting skills. While very few of us like to be tested, skills testing doesn't have to be a cause for panic. In this article, I'm going to write a bit about how to minimize test anxiety and do your best on formal assessments.

In my experience, people fail tests for one of three reasons:

1. They don't actually know the content or have the skills being tested.
2. They are confused by the test format.
3. They are so nervous about being tested that they can't demonstrate what they really know.

All three of these problems can be addressed by adequately preparing for a test. I'm always amazed at people who walk into interpreting tests without any preparation at all. No wonder the pass rate for the Federal Court Interpreter Exam is only 4%! So, here are some suggestions for preparing for an interpreting skills test that will actually stand you in good stead for any type of exam.

Investigate the test.

Well before your test date, find out all you can about what is on the test and how it will be administered. Any credible standardized test will have a preparation booklet that tells you about the test. While we don't know exactly what content will be included on a national interpreter certification, a review of the content of existing interpreter assessments gives us a clue. You will almost certainly be tested on:

- Knowledge of the National Code of Ethics
- Knowledge of the National Standards of Practice
- Healthcare terminology, both meaning and conversion
- Accurate consecutive interpreting, bidirectional

In addition, an interpreting test might assess:

- Accurate sight translation, bi-directional
- Simultaneous interpreting, bi-directional
- English grammar
- The ability to match register
- Written translation of very short texts
- Basic knowledge of healthcare concepts

In addition to asking what will be on the test, find out how the content will be tested. Interpreting tests almost always have a written portion and an oral portion. Will the written portion be multiple choice? Fill-in-the-blanks? Matching? Short answer? Labeling an anatomy diagram? Essay? And will the oral portion be recorded? Videotaped? Or rated live? Knowing what to expect in the testing process will make it easier to prepare before you go and to stay calm once you are there.

Study for the test.

Once you know what is going to be on the test, set up a study program. Read and reread the National Code of Ethics and Standards of Practice (you can download them for free from the website of the National Council on Interpreting in Health Care at www.ncihc.org) . Check out a self-study program on medical terminology, or read up on common health problems on websites like Medline Plus (www.medlineplus.gov). If you are an experienced medical interpreter, you may already know all you need to know for a national exam, but it never hurts to learn a little more.

Practice.

That preparation booklet from the testing organization will often contain practice exercises. **Do them.** Practice interpreting what you hear on the radio or TV. Sight-translate the newspaper. Take a look at the free medical brochures in your doctor's office and write down all the words you don't know. Buy tape sets such as ACEBO's *Interpreter's R_X* to practice with, or practice with friends. Translate prescriptions. If you are a working interpreter, you probably get a lot of practice already, but the more you can practice with someone who can catch your errors, the better prepared you'll be.

Sleep well the night before, and eat moderately before the exam.

Of course you are not going to do well on a test if you're so tired you doze off. In this country, most of us are chronically sleep deprived. So really try to get a full night's sleep the night before a big test. Eat before the test so that you'll have energy and not be distracted by a growling stomach, but don't overeat; too big a meal will make you sleepy and unable to think clearly.

Don't cram.

If you don't know it the night before the test, extra studying the morning of the test will not help. As a matter of fact, studies have shown that pressured studying right before a test actually distracts people and makes them do worse. So do your studying well in advance, over a period of weeks or months, not at the last minute.

When taking the test, read the questions carefully.

It's easy to get nervous on a test, especially on a timed test, and to feel you need to work quickly. That may be true, but careless reading of the question leads to giving the wrong answer. Read questions and instructions twice before answering, just to make sure you understand what is being asked.

If the test is timed, bring a watch.

Timed tests add pressure, that's for sure. So bring a watch, take it off your wrist and put it on your desk in front of you. You'll be more likely to see it there and be able to keep an eye on how you are doing relative to the clock. Most likely you will find you actually have more time than you think you do.

If the test is graded by machine, bring a ruler.

A standardized test being offered to many people has to graded by machine to be cost effective, so standardized tests often make use of an answer sheet consisting of the question's number followed by four "balloons," one corresponding to each multiple choice answer. The candidate must color in the balloon next to the correct answer. Do you know how many people fail these tests because they mess up filling in the balloon? So, make sure to fill in the circle completely, erase completely if you change your answer, and use a ruler to make sure that you are filling in the answer on the correct line. One line off, and all your answers will be wrong!

Skip questions you don't know, and come back to them.

Many timed tests are designed to have more questions than anyone can reasonably complete, as a means of allowing all candidates - even the best - to work to capacity. Of all those questions, you want to answer as many as you can. Since an answer left blank is counted as wrong, answer first the ones you know, then go back and work on the questions of which you are not sure. This way you will maximize the questions you get right.

If you absolutely don't know, guess.

Again, an answer left blank is wrong. If you really have no idea as to the correct answer, write down something; at least there is a chance you will be correct. If the test is being graded subjectively, this gives the grader some option of giving partial credit.

True and False questions:

True and false questions are those in which a statement is made and you must judge whether it is true or false. These questions are really frustrating, because the best answer is almost always "It depends." Unfortunately, "it depends" is never one of the options, so ask yourself, "Is this statement more true than false or more false than true?" In addition, when reading a true/false question, pay special attention to categorical words like *all, none, always, never*. These red-flag words almost always indicate that "false" is the correct answer.

Multiple choice tests:

Multiple choice questions usually have four possible answers from which you must choose the best. You will often find that two of the four are clearly wrong and two are reasonable. But which of the two is the correct answer? Remember that you are looking for the best answer, so both may be technically correct, but one may be more complete. Go back and read the question again carefully. And if you just don't know, guess; with only four answers, even a random guess has a 25% chance of being right.

Conclusion

By preparing carefully and using these little tricks, you can make sure that your results on an interpreter skills test are a true reflection of your skill level, and not a reflection of nerves or a lack of familiarity with the testing format. And with that – happy testing!

May 2009

37.

Interpreting with a Broken Heart

I guess I'll call him Antonio. That wasn't his real name, of course, but it will do. He was a handsome young man, early 20's, in prime physical condition, a nationally recognized athlete in his home country. He had always dreamed of coming to the U.S. to compete in his sport. He came instead for a bone marrow transplant to combat leukemia.

I only interpreted for Antonio and his family three times. The first time, for the initial meeting with the medical team, I couldn't believe he was even sick. He looked so healthy, so incredibly well! Weeks later, after chemotherapy had destroyed his bone marrow and steroids had wiped out his immune system, the change was a visceral shock to me. He was weak, his face grossly swollen from the medications. He could barely talk. The third and last time I interpreted for the family was the hardest. The purpose of the meeting was to impart the news to Antonio and, most of all to his family, that the transplant was not a success. The prognosis was bad. Antonio was expected to die. It was confirmed to me, quietly, by another interpreter on the team a few weeks later. Antonio was gone.

Death. Permanent disability. Disfigurement. Genetic defects. Chronic debilitating disease. Poor prognoses. The bad news that providers hate to give is the bad news that interpreters hate to interpret. And yet, it is part of health care, part of communication, and so, part of our work.

As an interpreter, how do you handle the imparting of bad news - both the interpretation itself and your own feelings about what is happening? It can be very difficult. Sometimes providers use vague euphemisms that English speakers would understand but which transfer poorly into other languages. Other times they are inappropriately blunt, telling patients things that culturally would never be told to them in their home country. Some cases are heartbreaking, and we want to help: somehow — but instead feel overwhelmed and distraught. What to do?

Every case is different and requires sensitivity and clarity of purpose. After talking with interpreters around the country about this issue, I was able to distill some suggestions that interpreters have found to be useful in dealing with these difficult situations.

How to handle the interpretation

The most important principle to keep in mind is: stay calm and focus on your purpose in the interaction. It is extremely important that you stay composed and focused, however sad or upset you may feel inside. You are there to facilitate understanding in communication between these people. You are of **no use** to the patient or his/her family if you fall apart. Indeed, you will make it more difficult for everyone involved if you do. Remember that you are this family's only link to the information that the provider is offering. You can cry when you get into your car or when you hang up the phone. While in the interaction, you have a job to do.

It may shock you just how the healthcare provider goes about imparting bad news to the family. Providers in the U.S. have been taught to be fairly direct in giving bad news, and this may be especially true of younger doctors. While common in health care in this country, it is often not the expectation of families who come from elsewhere. With your knowledge of the patient's culture, you may realize that the doctor's direct approach could be considered dangerously inappropriate by the patient and his family. In these cases, you **cannot** edit bad news to make it more palatable. However, you **can** discuss with the provider the cultural norms for giving bad news in the patient's culture.

If you simply cannot stay composed, or if the provider's insistence on giving bad news directly to the patient is in clear conflict with the family's express wish that such bad news not be given to the patient, you do have the option of withdrawing. Consider, however, that your withdrawal will require the session to be rescheduled or an ad-hoc interpreter to be brought in. Both of these options may lead to more pain and confusion for the patient and the family, so weigh carefully a decision to withdraw; it should not be taken lightly.

When the interpreting is over

When the interpreting session is over, you in-person interpreters may feel you'd like to say something to the family. Expressing condolences in a culturally appropriate manner is entirely acceptable, and will most likely be welcomed by the family. Be careful not to offer false hope, though, and do not initiate any physical contact (a hug, etc.). If a death has occurred, and if you feel you would like to attend the memorial service or funeral, this is also acceptable; many doctors, nurses and hospice workers do this for patients whom they have served for some time. If you choose to go further in expressing sympathy, however, and become a friend to the family, you are disqualifying yourself from interpreting for this family in the future.

How to handle your own feelings

It is natural and normal to feel sad after interpreting for a "bad news" session. Some interpreters are able to distance themselves from these feelings - to "not take their work home," as they say. However, most of us need to find ways to process our grief over what we've just witnessed. We need to find the manner and the time to grieve. Each of us will handle this in a different way; here are some ideas that interpreters included on a survey of how they deal with grief.

> "I talk to my husband about what happened, but I make sure never to include names or anything that could identify the patient. I just share the circumstances. He's very understanding, and that helps me."
>
> "I believe that when people die, they return to God, they're in a better place. I only had one patient who died. I lit a candle and said a prayer for his soul and asked God to be with the family. That made me feel like I'd done something for them, and it brought me comfort as well."
>
> "When I've had an interpreting session with bad news, I take some time to go walk in the woods later."
>
> "I work at a Children's Hospital, and some of the things I see just break my heart. Sometimes I cry in the car before driving home. But it makes me grateful too that my family doesn't suffer like that."
>
> "After bad news at work, I make a point to go out with my family and do something fun. It's like reminding myself that everything's not hopeless."

You will find your own way to deal with the sadness that comes with interpreting bad news. If you find, though, that a particular case is still weighing on your mind, and that you still feel generally sad weeks later, seek help. Some health care facilities provide on-site counseling for staff and may make it available to interpreters as well. If you are part of a faith community, the clergy may be of help. Talking to an interpreter services manager may also be useful. Don't ignore your feelings, though; patients and providers all need you to be emotionally healthy, as they all depend on you.

And that may be the most useful thing of all to remember. However hard hearing bad news may have been for a patient and family, your participation made it infinitely easier. Imagine Antonio and his family facing leukemia and then death without being able to communicate with Antonio's doctors. Imagine Antonio's little sister being pressed into interpreting because a professional interpreter wasn't there. As hard as interpreting for bad news is, the fact that you are there to facilitate communication helps. And who else but a professional interpreter would be able to keep interpreting even with a broken heart?

October, 2003

38.

A Christmas Poem for Interpreters

(Apologies to Clement Clarke Moore)

Twas the night before Christmas, and all through the house,
Not a creature was stirring, not even a mouse.
The teenagers sprawled all awry in their beds,
While visions of skateboards caromed in their heads.
And I with my headset and glossary too
Had just settled in for a session or two.
Telephonic interpreting seemed to make sense
To help pay a bit of the Christmas expense.

I'd picked up the phone and was just signing on
When something big zoomed by outside and was gone.
And up on the rooftop I heard such a noise,
I muted my microphone, really annoyed.
"Now what could that be?" I grumped, a bit irked,
"They know not to bother me when I'm at work.
"I'll just have to go check; I can see I'm committed.
"Background noise when interpreting isn't permitted."

I crept from my office and down the front stairs
And into the living room, not a bit scared,
When what from the fireplace suddenly appeared
But a man dressed in red with a fuzzy white beard.
The cap on this head and his bag did the trick;
I could tell in a moment this must be St. Nick.
But he didn't look jolly or jovial or cheery.
"Quick girl, do you speak any Reindeer?" he queried.

Now it happens that I, among other fine traits,
Am facile with languages, and I speak eight.
Among them - a secret not too many know -
Are Penguin and Reindeer and a smidgen of Crow
Which I learned one September when I was just two
And I got left behind at the Woodland Park Zoo.
(A wonderful place if you want to learn Trout;
But the wolves' accent I never could figure out.).

So there I was talking to jolly St. Nick
Who looked like he might be about to be sick.
"I need an interpreter! I'm in a stew.
"The reindeer won't fly. I don't know what to do!
"I need to find out what the problem could be,
"But I don't speak Reindeer, and they can't talk to me.
"I've shouted, used sign language, practically cried!"
"This sounds like a job for a pro" I replied.

The next thing I knew I was up on the roof
With the red-suited man and his reindeer to boot.
I did a quick pre-session, gave a small glance
And faded back in my interpreting stance.
It didn't take long, to old Santa's delight,
To learn that the elves had the harness too tight.
A terrible problem (but easily fixed)
When you're pulling a sleigh with a whole load of gifts.

The harness adjusted, the reindeer at ease,
St. Nick left some presents down under the tree.
Then he handed me one that he'd left till the end.
"And this is for you now, my bilingual friend,
"To thank you for saving our Christmas this year.

"What would we have done if you hadn't been here?"
Then I opened the box and I smiled to myself,
For I found here a bilingual gloss'ry of Elf.

We laughed and I wondered just how he had known
I'd been studying Elf late at night all alone.
He leaned close and said, "We sure need you around.
"Chief North Pole Interpreter – how does that sound?"
Then putting his finger aside of his nose,
He smiled and then up the chimney he rose.
And I heard him cry as he zoomed off with a streak,
"Merry Christmas to you all, whatever you speak!"

December 2006

Part 2

Exercises and Crossword Puzzles

Note: Crossword puzzles were created with the help of Puzzlemaker at DiscoveryEducation.com.

39.

The Vocabulary of Obstetrics
Terminology Exercise

This exercise, and the ones that follow, are designed to help interpreters expand both their understanding of particular areas of health care practice and their medical vocabulary in English.

This exercise is in obstetrics. I have tried to choose terminology that is neither too basic nor too technical. And men, don't think you're off the hook just because female interpreters are sent more often to obstetric appointments: you never know when it might be your turn in the delivery room!

There are two parts. First, see if you can match the terms with the definitions below. Then, using the same terms, fill in the blanks in the narrative that follows.

Terms

_______ abortion

_______ miscarriage

_______ Rh factor

_______ Down syndrome

_______ bag of waters

_______ epidural

_______ cesarean section

_______ fetal distress

_______ fetal monitor

_______ breech presentation

_______ natural childbirth

_______ alpha fetoprotein

_______ dilated

_______ umbilical cord

_______ preeclampsia

_______ episiotomy

_______ let-down reflex

_______ meconium

_______ amniocentesis

_______ inverted nipples

_______ Corionic Villus Sampling (CVS)

_______ crowning

_______ afterbirth

Definitions

1. An adverse condition of the fetus, often identified by the excessively rapid or slow fetal heart tones or by the passage of meconium in utero.
2. A device that measures a fetus' heart rate.
3. The first proteins that form the basis of blood in an embryo. When found to be elevated in amniotic fluid, they can be a sign of fetal anencephaly (lack of a brain) or open neural tube defects such as spina bifida.
4. An antigen that may or may not be found on human blood cells. If it is present in the mother and not in the fetus (or vice versa), the mother's body may mount an immune response that can result in the over-thickening of the fetus' blood and fetal death.
5. The thick greenish-black material found in the intestines of a full-term fetus. It constitutes the first stools passed by a newborn.
6. Induced termination of a pregnancy.

7. A toxic condition including high blood pressure (hypertension), protein in the urine (proteinuria), and swelling (edema), due to pregnancy; it can lead to convulsions and coma.
8. A genetic disorder associated with an extra 21st chromosome.
9. A surgical incision into the perineum and vagina to prevent tearing during delivery.
10. A method for diagnosis of fetal diseases by sampling the cells of the placenta for DNA analysis.
11. A spontaneous expulsion of the fetus from the womb before the completion of gestation.
12. The amniotic sac.
13. The injection of a local anesthetic into the space around the lumbar spinal cord in order to numb the lower half of the body.
14. A surgical incision of the walls of the abdomen and uterus for delivery of a fetus.
15. A method for diagnosis of fetal diseases by sampling the fluid in the amniotic sac for DNA analysis.
16. The turning inward of the nipples.
17. A cord arising from the fetus's navel that connects the fetus with the placenta and contains the two umbilical arteries and the umbilical vein.
18. When the baby emerges from the birth canal bottom first.
19. An involuntary reflex during breast feeding that allows the milk to flow freely.
20. A stage in childbirth when the top of the fetus' head emerges from the vulva.
21. A system of managing childbirth in which the mother receives preparatory education in order to remain conscious during, and assist in delivery with minimal or no use of drugs or anesthetics.
22. Enlarged, stretched.
23. The placenta and fetal membranes that are expelled after delivery.

Fill-in Exercise

Now see if you can fit the words into the appropriate sentence. Verbs may be conjugated to fit the sense of the sentence.

Mrs. Green was pleased when she found out she was pregnant again. She had already had two ________________ (one at six weeks and one at three months), and she was a bit afraid that she might not be able to carry to term. She was also a bit surprised that her obstetrician wanted her to have a series of tests, just because she was 38 years old. The first was just a blood test to check for ________________, which turned out normal. But when an ultrasound showed nucal thickening, the doctor suggested that she have a ________________ to rule out ________________. This test showed some abnormalities, but the doctor explained that it might just be the placenta that was affected. So Mrs. Green went back at 14 weeks for an ________________. Thank goodness that test came back normal! She also learned that her ________________ was the same as the baby's, which was a relief. Blood tests ruled out gestational diabetes and blood pressure checks ruled out ________________.

It was early in the morning, four days before her due date, when Mrs. Green felt her ________________ break. She and her family all went to the hospital. The doctor checked her cervix and found that she was only three centimeters dilated, so she had a while to wait. Over the following hours labor progressed slowly. Mrs. Green had prepared for ________________ and wanted no drugs or anesthesia, but as the hours wore on, she became very tired. Her obstetrician hooked her up to a ________________ to see how she and the baby were doing.

After 12 hours of labor, Mrs. Green had dilated to ten centimeters and was finally ready to deliver. The obstetrician did an ________________ so that Mrs. Green's perineum would not tear during delivery. Then, as the baby entered the birth canal and started to ________________, the ________________ suddenly showed the baby entering into ________________. A resident who was there suggested giving Mrs. Green an ________________ and doing an emergency ________________ to remove the baby surgically. The obstetrician however, carefully supporting the baby's head, inserted a finger into the birth canal and found that the ________________ was wrapped around the baby's neck. She slipped it over the baby's head, and the baby was quickly born.

A few minutes later, the ____________________ was delivered, and a nurse placed Mrs. Green's new baby girl on her breast. Even though her milk wouldn't ____________________ for a while, the baby latched right on and started sucking. The family came in to visit and see their new daughter and sister for the first time.

The Real Test

The real test of an interpreter is the ability to transmit meaning from one language to another. Obstetrics is filled with terms that have a multitude of regionally-specific equivalents. The preceding exercises are designed to help you understand the terminology in English; now see if you can find either a direct linguistic equivalent or a way to clearly and succinctly explain the term in your non-English language. If you speak a language with a great deal of regional variation (such as Spanish or Arabic), see if you can come up with a number of different equivalents. Then practice sight translating the preceding exercise into your non-English language until your command of the key vocabulary is complete.

> There are many useful sites on the internet to look up medical terminology. Here's one I like:
> http://medical-dictionary.com
> It's easy to use and provides definitions written for the general public, not for medical specialists.

April 2005

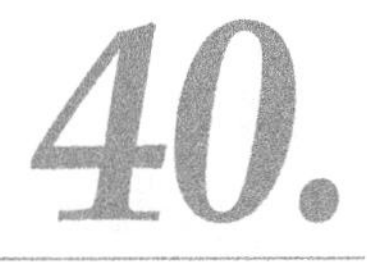

The Vocabulary of Housing Services

Terminology Exercise

This exercise is concerned with Social Service's terminology. However, since Social Services encompass a wide range of venues, we'll narrow it down a bit and focus on housing issues.

See if you can match the following housing terms with the definitions below.[1]

Terms

_______ application fee

_______ transitional housing

_______ reinstate

_______ credit check

_______ evaluation

_______ eligible

_______ low-income

_______ vacancy

_______ Section 8 housing

_______ 30-day notice

_______ case manager

_______ referral

_______ security deposit

_______ annual review

_______ lease

_______ subsidized

_______ evict

_______ inspection

_______ voucher

_______ food stamps

_______ grievance hearing

_______ tax-credit apartment

_______ Housing Authority

_______ pay-or-vacate notice

Definitions:

1. To force a tenant to leave a rented apartment/house by legal action.
2. A person working for a social services agency who helps a client work on goal areas.
3. Money paid to a landlord to reimburse for any damage to the property found after a tenant leaves.
4. A monthly monetary grant from the government that the recipient may use to buy food.
5. Money that is paid when an application is submitted to pay for processing the application.
6. A government organization that administers low-income housing in a certain city or county.
7. A process done before occupancy to make sure the rental property is in good condition.
8. The first legal warning before an eviction.

---

[1] Many thanks to the staff of the Seattle YWCA for help with the definitions.

9. A Federal Government program allowing tenants to pay only 30% of their income for rent.
10. Household income under the national poverty line.
11. To put back in place benefits that have been removed.
12. When part of the cost of some service or expense is paid by the government.
13. Temporary housing, usually with case management services.
14. An unoccupied residence.
15. The paperwork assuring rental subsidy or other services.
16. The process of re-evaluating a case after one year has passed.
17. A legal document governing the rental of a property.
18. A process done before renting to a prospective tenant that allows the landlord to see the financial history of the tenant.
19. Meeting the criteria to receive some benefit.
20. A legal proceeding in which an individual can protest an action by a government entity.
21. A legal notice that a tenant has 30 days to vacate a property.
22. Paperwork that transfers an individual's case from one agency to another.
23. A program created by Congress that allows the tenant to pay only 30% of the area median income as reported by the Department of Housing and Urban Development (HUD).
24. An assessment.

Fill-in exercise:

Now see if you can fit the words into the appropriate sentence. Remember, verbs may be conjugated to fit the sense of the sentence.

Fatana couldn't find a place to live. It seemed that everywhere she looked, the rents were too expensive. Even with her ________________ from the WIC program to help pay for food, she couldn't seem to find enough money to pay for an apartment. And the process of finding an apartment for herself and her family was so complicated! Finally, a social worker gave her a ________________ to the ________________.

The Housing Authority helps ________________ families find a place to live by helping them apply to the government for ________________, for ________________, or for other ________________ housing programs. They often help people who are moving back into general society from ________________.

After an assessment of Fatana's situation, the Housing Authority determined that she was ________________ to receive assistance. With help from her ________________, Fatana learned about how the housing market works. First she had to wait for a ________________ in Section 8 Housing. When an apartment was finally available, the landlord then asked Fatana to fill out an application and to pay an ________________. Then he did a ________________ to see how well Fatana had paid her bills in the past. Once he had approved her application and had reviewed her ________________, Fatana had to pay a ________________ on the apartment; she was told that if she took good care of the apartment, she'd get this back later. She and the landlord did an ________________ of the property together, so they would both agree on the condition of the property before she moved in. The landlord asked her to sign a rental agreement (called a ________________) and explained that she would need to pay her rent on time. If she repeatedly failed to pay her rent, he would send her a ________________. If she still did not pay, he would send her a ________________, informing her that he was starting the legal proceedings to have her ________________.

After a year, Fatana had an ________________ and was shocked when she found that the Housing Authority intended to terminate her benefits. She immediately requested a ____________________ to protest her loss of benefits. The Housing Authority did an ____________________ of her case, and, realizing that they had made a mistake, they ____________________ her in the program.

The Real Test

As with vocabulary in many specialty areas, the vocabulary of Social Services often has no easily understood linguistic equivalent. The preceding exercises are designed to help you understand the terminology in English; now see if you can find either a direct linguistic equivalent or a way to clearly and succinctly explain the term in your non-English language. Then practice sight translating the preceding exercise into your non-English language until your command of the key vocabulary is complete.

July 2004

41.

The Vocabulary of Domestic Abuse

Terminology Exercise

This is another exercise designed to help interpreters in health care expand both their understanding of particular areas of practice and their medical vocabulary in English. Here, our focus is on the vocabulary commonly used in Social Services when dealing with domestic violence.

First, see if you can match the following terms with the definitions that follow. Then, using the same terms, fill in the blanks in the narrative.

Terms:

_______ advocate

_______ Child Protective Services (CPS)

_______ safety plan

_______ crisis line

_______ cycle of abuse

_______ domestic violence

_______ goals and objectives

_______ intimate partner

_______ protection order

_______ victim

_______ confidential

_______ TANF (Temporary Aid for Needy Families)

_______ to file for dissolution

_______ confidential shelter

_______ communal setting

_______ survivor

_______ crazy-making

_______ red flags

_______ walking on eggshells

_______ abuser

_______ put-downs

_______ shelter

_______ transitional housing program

Definitions:

1. The person committing abuse or violence against another in a relationship.
2. The job title of the women that work in the shelter. Their job is helping shelter clients help themselves.
3. A living arrangement in which a group of unrelated people share a house and everyone shares the work to keep the house running smoothly (chores, cooking, meals etc).
4. Information that should not be shared with others; private.
5. The agency of the government that responds to / investigates reports of child abuse.
6. Behavior by an intimate partner that makes you feel like you're going crazy; for example, hiding your car keys.
7. Repetitive behavior of abuse.
8. Fill out the legal paperwork asking for the termination of a marriage.
9. Abuse by one intimate partner of another intimate partner.

10. The specific way in which a woman wants the shelter to help her.
11. The member of an adult (romantic) relationship (husband/wife, boyfriend/girlfriend, or parents of the same child).
12. A court order directing one person (the abuser) not to have contact with or hurt another person (the victim). If the abuser violates the order by contacting or hurting the victim, he/she can be arrested.
13. Indicators that someone is abusive.
14. An abused women's plan to keep herself safe from being abused or seeing her abuser if she does not want to.
15. A safe house where women and children can go to live temporarily, if they need to leave their homes because of violence or abuse.
16. Cash and food benefits from the government.
17. Low income housing where a resident can stay temporarily, usually for 6-18 months.
18. A telephone number that a victim of abuse can call to get help fast.
19. When a woman feels as if she needs to be extremely careful in everything she says and does so as not to trigger the abuser into violent behavior.
20. Insults.
21. A person who is still suffering in an abusive relationship.
22. A person who has gotten out of an abusive relationship.
23. A shelter whose address is given only to those who are going to stay there or who are providing services there.

Fill-in exercise:

Now see if you can fit the words into the appropriate sentence. Remember, verbs may be conjugated to fit the sense of the sentence.

Alba was afraid for her life and for the lives of her children. Alba's husband, Raúl, was a violent man. He had hit both her and her children in the past, and this time he had beaten her up so badly that she'd had to go to the hospital. When she was released, she was afraid to go home. She was so tired of ___________________, always afraid that something she said might trigger Raúl's violent temper. Even worse, she was afraid that he might start to hit the children, and that the State Office of ___________________ might take the children away. She was fed up with being a ___________________, accepting anything that Raúl did to her.

So instead of going home, Alba picked up the telephone and called a ___________________. The person who answered the phone was trained to help people who were having personal emergencies. This person told Alba about Domestic Abuse Women's Network (DAWN). DAWN is a ___________________ for women and children who are victims of ___________________. That means that their ___________________ abuse them physically and/or psychologically. The people who work at DAWN help women break the ___________________ by assisting them in becoming independent of the abuser, in becoming ___________________ instead of victims.

When Alba got to the DAWN shelter, she felt safe for the first time in years. This was a ___________________; nobody could even get the address unless they actually worked there or needed help there. Alba met with an ___________________ who helped Alba develop ___________________ about what she wanted to happen. This person also helped her develop a ___________________ for herself and her children so that she would always know how to keep them and herself safe. Her advocate helped Alba file for a ___________________ (also called a "restraining order" or a "no-contact order"), so that Raúl could not come near her or her children. She also helped Alba apply to the State Medicaid office for ___________________, so that she'd have some income, and to a ___________________, so that she could find her own place to live.

At DAWN, Alba lived in a __________________, together with other women who's been abused and their children. She felt safe there, especially because everything she told her advocate was kept __________________, even from the other women at the shelter. She could decide what and when she wanted other people to know about her situation. She did share some things in her women's group, where she learned about the __________________ that indicate that a man may be an __________________. She learned that abuse is more than just physical violence. It includes all the constant __________________ she got from Raúl and the __________________ things her husband did on purpose just to make her feel bad. She began to think about whether she should end her marriage by __________________.

The Real Test

As I mentioned previously, the real test of an interpreter is the ability to transmit meaning from one language to another. As with vocabulary in many specialty areas, the vocabulary of Social Services often has no easily understood linguistic equivalent. The preceding exercises are designed to help you understand the terminology in English; now see if you can find either a direct linguistic equivalent or a way to clearly and succinctly explain the term in your non-English language. Then practice sight translating the preceding exercise into your non-English language until your command of the key vocabulary is complete.

August 2004

42.

The Vocabulary of Dentistry

Terminology Exercise

The subject of this chapter is the vocabulary of dentistry.

Some of you may be thinking that you don't get called much for dental appointments. But here's an interesting thought: many dental offices are starting to use telephonic interpreting, specifically because they need an interpreter only for the short consults before and after they work on the patient. And if you think dental vocabulary is a snap, think again. Many of the terms are common words that have specific meanings in the dental context. So, "pulp" is not the stuff that comes in orange juice, and "calculus" is not that what you studied in math class; "plaque" isn't something you hang on your wall, and "recession" isn't what's happening to the economy. For clear communication, it's important to learn the terminology.

Terms:

______ dental floss

______ calculus

______ extract

______ wisdom tooth

______ decay

______ plaque

______ bite

______ periodontal disease

______ milk teeth

______ pulp

______ crowding

______ overbite

______ gums

______ gingivitis

______ bridge

______ prophylaxis

______ root canal

______ palate

______ impacted

______ cavity

______ braces

______ orthodontist

______ retainer

______ dentures

______ sealants

______ fluoride

______ recession

______ abscess

______ enamel

______ crown

Definitions

1. The way the teeth meet.
2. The hole that runs through the center of the root where the pulp is; a treatment to clear out this area and putting a filling in it, when the pulp is damaged.
3. A hole in the tooth caused by decay.
4. The tissue that covers the jawbone and surrounds the teeth.
5. All the changes that occur in a tooth that is attacked by caries.
6. Plastic coatings for teeth.
7. The hard outer layer of the teeth.
8. A chemical present in food and often added to water that strengthens the teeth.
9. A gum disease around the edges of the gum next to the teeth, caused

by not properly cleaning the teeth.

10. What happens to a tooth if it does not have room to erupt normally and ends up jammed against another tooth or trapped inside the bone.
11. The first set of teeth that a child gets; baby teeth.
12. A dentist who specializes in the moving of teeth using braces.
13. An infection.
14. The distance that the upper front teeth come down over the lower front teeth.
15. An artificial tooth that is fitted over a natural tooth when the natural tooth is broken or decayed.
16. The roof of the mouth.
17. Gum disease.
18. Thread for cleaning between the teeth.
19. A sticky layer of germs and very small bits of food that builds up over the teeth.
20. Hard deposits on the teeth; hardened plaque.
21. Cleaning of the teeth, by removing plaque and polishing the teeth.
22. Not enough space to fit all the teeth evenly.
23. The nerve of the tooth, together will blood vessels and connective tissues.
24. False teeth that can be removed.
25. A condition where the gum pulls back from the tooth.
26. The springs, wires and brackets that are put on the teeth to move the teeth into a different position.
27. To remove a tooth.
28. A type of brace put in after teeth have been moved, to hold them in the right place.
29. False teeth that are permanently stuck to the natural teeth.
30. The third molar.

Fill-in exercise:

Now see if you can fit the words into the appropriate sentence. Not all the words will be used, and some will be used twice.

Good morning, Mrs. Hong. I'm Dr. Nguyen. Before we get going on your children's cleaning, I'd like to let you know what we'll be doing today.

Mainly, we'll be doing ____________________ on the children today, to make sure their teeth are nice and clean and to get rid of any ____________________ and ____________________. Then I'll take a look in their mouths, just to check for possible ____________________. We'll apply a ____________________ treatment, to protect the ____________________ on the teeth, and on the two older children, we'll also be putting ____________________ on their molars to protect against ____________________.

Now, about your youngest daughter, May; I see that her ____________________ are beginning to fall out and that she's getting her adult teeth. There seems to be a fair bit of ____________________, so I think you should be prepared that she will probably need ____________________ when she's a bit older to straighten the teeth out and to correct her ____________________. I'll refer you to an ____________________ when the time comes. We'll probably want to ____________________ her ____________________ too, when they start to come in, since there probably won't be enough room for them. Unless they are ____________________, that's a fairly simple procedure.

Now let's talk about your dental needs for a moment. First of all, the X-rays showed that there is a very deep ____________________ in this tooth here and that the pulp has become badly infected. It's beginning to form an ____________________. I'll bet that hurts a lot. We're going to need to do a ____________________, but first I'd like to treat the infection with an antibiotic. After we clean out the ____________________, control the infection and do the ____________________, I'll put a ____________________ on the tooth.

Secondly, I can see that you're getting some ____________________ of the ____________________ – see here where the root of the tooth is beginning to show? You can stop this process by a using ____________________ every day. That will also help you lower your risk here of ____________________.

Finally, I see you're missing a tooth back here. As a result, the neighboring teeth are shifting out of their correct placement. Have you thought about getting a ____________________? That would help the teeth stay in the right place.

The Real Test

And, you know what's coming next. Can you express these English terms in your non-English language? Go get your bilingual dictionary and see if you can find either a direct linguistic equivalent or a way to clearly and succinctly explain the term in your non-English language. Then practice sight translating the preceding exercise into your non-English language until your command of the key vocabulary is complete. This homework will really give you something to sink your teeth into!

October 2004

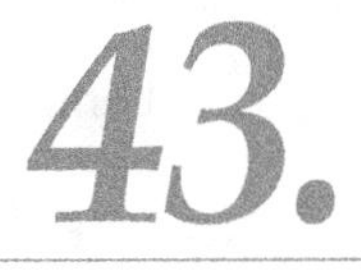

The Vocabulary of the Business Office

Terminology Exercise

This is another exercise designed to help interpreters in health care expand both their understanding of particular areas of health care practice and their medical vocabulary in English. This chapter's topic is the vocabulary of the hospital financial office.

Terms:

_______ occupation

_______ spouse

_______ insurance

_______ policy

_______ work-related injury

_______ medical record

_______ next-of-kin

_______ benefits

_______ co-pay

_______ deductible

_______ eligible

_______ coinsurance

_______ retroactive

_______ advanced directive

_______ appeal

_______ pre-existing condition

_______ certificate of coverage

_______ COBRA

_______ Federal Poverty Level

_______ fee-for-service

_______ low income

_______ Medicaid

_______ Medicare

_______ managed care

_______ partner

_______ WIC (Women, Infants and Children)

_______ power of attorney

_______ primary care provider

_______ prior authorization review

_______ SSI (Supplemental Security Income)

Definitions

1. Document specifying the terms, coverage and cost of an insurance plan.
2. Poor; earning little money.
3. A federal grant program that provides supplemental food, health care referrals and nutrition education to pregnant women, new mothers and their infants.
4. A physician, Physician's Assistant or Nurse Practitioner who is responsible for providing initial care and for supervising and coordinating all the care for a patient.
5. An approach to the provision of health care which integrates clinical care and administration into one system in which a primary care provider coordinates a patient's access to service.

6. Services offered by a program, an insurer, or a provider under a particular contract.
7. A federal income assistance program for needy individuals over 65 years of age, and for blind and disabled persons.
8. The amount of a person's health care bills that he must pay before the insurance company will start to pay.
9. Proof of coverage under a particular insurance policy.
10. A class of work: for example: lawyer, dishwasher, interpreter.
11. A file that contains the medical history of a patient.
12. The amount of money, in addition to what the insurance company will cover, that a patient must pay at the time of service in order to receive services.
13. Meeting the criteria to receive some benefit.
14. A legal document that authorizes one person to make decisions on behalf of another.
15. In questions of civil status, a person with whom one has an intimate relationship, who is not one's spouse.
16. A legal process to request that an official decision be reconsidered.
17. Husband or wife.
18. Guidelines issued every year by the federal government as a measure of poverty; often used to determine eligibility for certain federal programs.
19. A medical problem that had been identified before a patient joined a particular health plan.
20. A federal law that requires an employer to offer continued health insurance coverage to employees for up to 18 months after terminating employment.
21. A federally-funded program to provide medical benefits to persons over 65 years of age and certain disabled individuals.
22. Closest living relative.
23. Including something that came before.
24. A legal document created by an individual that states his wishes regarding certain aspects of medical care; this document is used in the case that the patient's health precludes him stating his preferences for himself. This document often details a person's preferences for end-of-life care.
25. The percentage of a health care bill that is the responsibility of the insured to pay, when the insurance plan covers less than 100% of allowable charges.
26. The process of getting approval for a specific health care procedure or medication before it is initiated.

27. A contract under which one party must pay for loss by another party.
28. A federally-funded program to provide medical benefits for certain low-income individuals.
29. A payment arrangement in which the patient is responsible for paying the full cost of his care.
30. A trauma that occurred while the injured person was at work.

Exercise

On the next page is a sample of a form frequently used in the hospitals, containing business terminology. First, see if you can express the English terms above in your non-English language. Then practice sight translating the Patient Registration Form into your non-English language until your command of the key vocabulary is complete.

Patient Registration Form

Medical Record Number: __________

Name (last, first, middle initial): ______________________________
Mailing Address: ______________________________
Residential Address: ______________________________
Telephone (w): ______________________________
Telephone (h): ______________________________
Social Security Number: ______________________________
Date of birth: ______________________________
Occupation: ______________________________
Employer: ______________________________

Marital status: ___ married ___ single ___ divorced ___ widowed ___ domestic partner
Spouse's name: ______________________________
Spouse's occupation: ______________________________
Spouse's employer: ______________________________
Emergency contact: ______________________________
Next of kin: ______________________________

Financial coverage
____ Self-pay
____ Commercial insurance: policy number ________________________
____ Medicaid
____ Medicare

Is this a work-related injury? ___ Yes ___ No

Have you filed an advanced directive with your primary care provider? ___ Yes ___ No
If not, you must do so within 24 hours of admission to the hospital.

NOTE:
If you are not eligible for Medicaid, Medicare, COBRA; and if your income (including SSI) is less than 200% of the Federal Poverty level; you may qualify for our discount payment program. This program requires only a small co-pay and has neither coinsurance nor deductible; nor can benefits be denied participation due to a pre-existing condition. You will have to show proof of income to qualify. If you are denied participation, you have the right to appeal, and if your appeal is successful, your costs will be covered retroactively.

November 2004

44.

Idioms, Acronyms & Abbreviations

Terminology Exercise

Holey moley, it's "that" time of the month again: time to take a gander at yet another big stumbling block for interpreters. And this month's challenge is interpreting idioms, acronyms and abbreviations.

Health related discourse is full of all three of these. Providers often use informal speech replete with idiomatic expressions to build rapport (or "break the ice") with patients. I remember one provider for whom I used to interpret who was famous among the interpreter staff for starting each session by looking at the patient and asking, "So-o-o, what's cookin'?" It was nice and friendly and all, but certainly posed a challenge to the interpreter!

Other idioms are more medically related. Patients in the ED get moved "onto the floor," parents of kids with fever are asked to "push fluids," overweight patients with high blood pressure are "a time bomb ticking." This colorful language is highly descriptive, but, again, hard to interpret.

Acronyms are those words made up of the first letters in a series of words. So Sudden Infant Death Syndrome becomes SIDS and the Department of Social and Health Services is DSHS. In the dominant culture's rush to speed everything up – even speech– this verbal shorthand allows people who share subject knowledge to save time when talking to each other. On the other hand, trying to understand acronym-laden speech when one doesn't share the same frame of reference can make one's head spin.

Abbreviations in several forms are also finding their way into our speech to a greater degree. Some are used as a written shorthand on forms ("lbs." for "pounds" or "m.i." for "middle initial"), but there is also a trend toward abbreviating some spoken terms. "Medications" are becoming "meds" and "laboratory tests" are often referred to as "labs."

How do we handle these linguistic boondoggles? Pretty much the same as we do all interpreting.

1. **Hear** the message (idiom / acronym / abbreviation) in the source language.
2. Extract the **meaning** (or ASK of you don't know).
3. Recreate the **meaning** in the target language. This may mean employing an idiom or acronym in the target language, or it may mean substituting a phrase that means the same.

The key to all this, of course, is understanding the idiom or acronym or abbreviation in the source language. Reading is a great way to expand your knowledge of idiomatic speech. Asking for explanation is another. And if you get stuck, here are some online resources that might be helpful:

- http://www.usingenglish.com/reference/idioms/a.html
- http://www.idiomsite.com
- http://idioms.thefreedictionary.com/
- http://www.medindia.net/acronym

So, don't be a stick in the mud! Spice up your speech with some idioms! Don't let your sense of humor go AWOL, and just lol when some provider starts using this abbreviated speech.

But make sure your interpretations are clear and accurate.

Exercise

Below you will find a list of English idioms and acronyms. If an idiom with the same meaning exists in your non-English language write it in the blank provided, in your non-English language.

If there is no idiom that conveys the same meaning in your non-English language, use the blank to explain the meaning of the idiom as you would if you were in an interpreting situation. You may do this in English.

Idioms

1. above all ___________
2. as fit as a fiddle ___________
3. as good as gold ___________
4. as hungry as a bear ___________
5. as regular as clockwork ___________
6. as sharp as a tack ___________
7. as sick as a dog ___________
8. baloney ___________
9. to beat around the bush ___________
10. bed of roses ___________
11. to break the ice ___________
12. a breeze ___________
13. bushed ___________
14. come rain or shine ___________
15. to cost an arm and a leg ___________
16. down the drain ___________
17. to eat like a horse ___________
18. fair and square ___________
19. to feel blue ___________
20. for the time being ___________
21. forty winks ___________
22. get a kick out of something (or someone) ___________
23. to go bananas ___________
24. to give the green light ___________
25. in a nutshell ___________
26. in a pickle ___________
27. in seventh heaven ___________
28. in the nick of time ___________
29. in the same boat ___________
30. ins and outs ___________
31. to keep the ball rolling ___________
32. the last straw ___________
33. a long face ___________
34. to make a mountain out of a molehill ___________
35. to nip something in the bud ___________
36. no dice ___________
37. on pins and needles ___________
38. on the ball ___________
39. on the fence ___________
40. on the house ___________

41. once in a blue moon ______________________
42. out of the blue ______________________
43. out of the woods ______________________
44. pain in the neck ______________________
45. to pan out ______________________
46. a piece of cake ______________________
47. to pull someone's leg ______________________
48. to put the cards on the table ______________________
49. to put two and two together ______________________
50. red tape ______________________
51. to run in the family ______________________
52. second nature ______________________
53. to see eye to eye ______________________
54. sink or swim ______________________
55. sixth sense ______________________
56. spick-and-span ______________________
57. to take pains ______________________
58. the tip of the iceberg ______________________
59. under the weather ______________________
60. a white lie ______________________

Medical Acronyms

61. AIDS ______________________
62. AMA ______________________
63. BM ______________________
64. BMI ______________________
65. CABG ______________________
66. CT (as in CT Scan) ______________________
67. CBC ______________________
68. COPD ______________________
69. ECG ______________________
70. EEG ______________________
71. EMG ______________________
72. GERD ______________________
73. GVHD ______________________
74. HIV ______________________
75. HPV ______________________
76. IUD ______________________
77. IVP ______________________
78. MI ______________________
79. MRI ______________________

80. NICU ______________________________
81. NPO ______________________________
82. NSAID ______________________________
83. PCP ______________________________
84. Rx ______________________________
85. Tx ______________________________
86. URI ______________________________
87. UTI ______________________________

Language Access Acronyms

88. OCR ______________________________
89. CHIA ______________________________
90. DHHS ______________________________
91. DOJ ______________________________
92. IMIA ______________________________
93. IS ______________________________
94. LAC ______________________________
95. LEP ______________________________
96. LLD ______________________________
97. NCIHC ______________________________
98. OPI ______________________________
99. ATA ______________________________
100. __________ The acronym of the interpreter association in your state.

December 2007

45.

Slang Vocabulary & Expressions

Terminology Exercise

This exercise, by popular demand, is on American slang. You've probably noticed that we native speakers of American English speak very differently than we write. Often slang is used the make an interaction less formal and more friendly. Still, slang can represent a real challenge to interpreters when it is introduced into health care interactions.

On the next page you'll find a series of slang expressions. See if you can match them to their meaning. (And, by the way, if you're really into American slang, then take a gander at the down-and-dirty website at www.urbandictionary.com, where you'll find some slang that's really over the top!)

Terms

_______ ahead of the game

_______ back to square one

_______ to backfire

_______ bang for the buck

_______ bells and whistles

_______ to bite the bullet

_______ to buy time

_______ to call the shots

_______ catch-22

_______ check it out

_______ to have a close call

_______ to cut down on

_______ give us a ring

_______ to go through channels

_______ goofed

_______ hop up here

_______ I take it

_______ lickety-split

_______ to pull something off

_______ to rule out

_______ to run in the family

_______ to slip on

_______ tah-dah!

_______ X marks the spot

Definitions[2]

1. A directive that is impossible to obey without violating some other, equally important directive.
2. Call us on the telephone.
3. Climb up on top of something.
4. To discard as a possibility.
5. Fancy gadgets.
6. Having an advantage in a competitive situation.
7. I understand.
8. Look at this.
9. Made a mistake.
10. To make something happen.
11. To make the decisions, be in charge.
12. To put on.
13. Quickly.
14. To be true for various family members.

---

[2] The definitions of terms in this exercise were taken from Spears, Richard A., NTC'S Dictionary of American slang and Colloquial Expressions. NTC Publishing Group, Chicago, 2000. 560 pages.

15. This is the exact place.
16. To accept something difficult and try to live with it.
17. To address a problem by going to the right person.
18. To barely escape something.
19. To examine something.
20. To get the opposite result of the one that was planned.
21. To have to start over again.
22. To use a tactic to postpone something.
23. To use less of.
24. Value for the effort or money spent.

Now see if you can fit the words into the appropriate sentence. (Hint: the verbs that are in the infinitive form above ["to" form] may be conjugated in the sentence.)

Mr. Sanchez, I know you don't want people to think you're disabled, but you're just going to have to ______________ and use a cane.

We should have the results next week. Why don't you ______________ and I'll go over them with you?

We thought that telling your Mom that she needs to do her exercises so that you all don't have to come take care of her every day would get her motivated, but the plan ____________; now she won't even try to do the exercises!

Let me give you a prescription for the 800 mg. pills instead of the 200 mg. They have ______________.

You are so lucky – you're getting the newest birthing suite in the hospital. It's got all the ______________.

This treatment isn't going to cure the cancer, but it will ______ us _________. (Hint: This sentence uses one phrase broken in the middle.)

We were going to wait to start the next round of chemotherapy, but you've responded so well so far that we're planning on starting next week. That way we'll be ______________.

I need to ask what your parents died of, because some health problems ______________.

You're stuck in a real ______________. If you go back to work, you'll lose your Medicaid, but if you don't go back to work, you won't be able to afford the co-pay for your services here. I'm not sure what to advise you!

I can only give you my opinion, Mrs. Nguyen; you and your family are the ones who are ______________.

Here on the ultrasound, you can see your baby, Mrs. Gorchenko. Hey, ______________, here's her little foot!

I need you to tell me exactly where your knee hurts, so tell me if it hurts as I press here. . . or here. . . or here. . or – ah hah! ______________!

It's a good thing you brought him in when you did. He was bleeding heavily internally. It was a ______________. Any later and I don't think we could have saved him.

Regarding your diet, you absolutely must _______________ the amount of salt you're eating. It's not good for your blood pressure.

I don't know if the hospital will give you a discount or not. We'll have to _______________ and see what they say.

Oops, I _______________.

Let's get that cast right off, and we'll have you out of here _______________.

All the tests came back negative. As far as figuring out what you have, we're _______________.

We usually don't use the laparoscope to do the surgery when the patient is in the middle of a gall bladder attack, but we gave it a try and we _______________.

This test will help us _______________ the possibility that the lump is cancer.

So, _______________ you don't feel the medication helped any.

Why don't you just _______________ this gown and _______________ on the exam table so that I can take a look at that shoulder? (Hint: This sentence uses two different phrases.)

So, we take the bandages off and --_______________! You can see!

June 2004

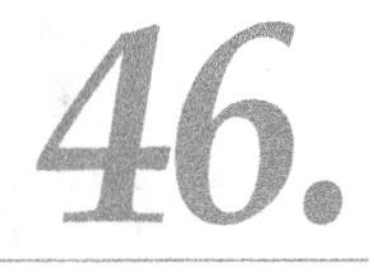

Signs & Symptoms

Crossword Puzzle

This exercise is on signs and symptoms, and to make it more fun, it takes the form of a crossword puzzle. Look at each clue, find the spaces (either across or down) that correspond to it, and find a word that fits. Good luck! And when you're done, try translating the words into your non-English language.

Across

2. Painful
5. A feeling of lightheadedness
6. To shake all over
8. "Grand mal" and "petite mal" are types of this
10. Unable to have a bowel movement
13. A lack of energy
16. Tic
17. Sad
19. A type of cough common with asthma
21. Unable to bend easily
22. An abnormally high temperature
23. Excess air in the stomach or colon
25. Not strong
26. Suppuration
28. Painful muscle contractions
29. Frequent watery stools

Down

1. When your voice gets lower and scratchy, it gets ____________.
3. Tinnitus
4. With no feeling
7. Watery mucus in the nostrils
9. A sense that the room is spinning around
11. Makes you want to scratch
12. Pins and needles
14. When small dry pieces of skin come off
15. To tremble, often from the cold
18. Acid backing up into the esophagus causes this
20. A migraine is one of these
24. Throwing up
26. Too early
27. How you feel before you lose consciousness
30. An irritation of the skin

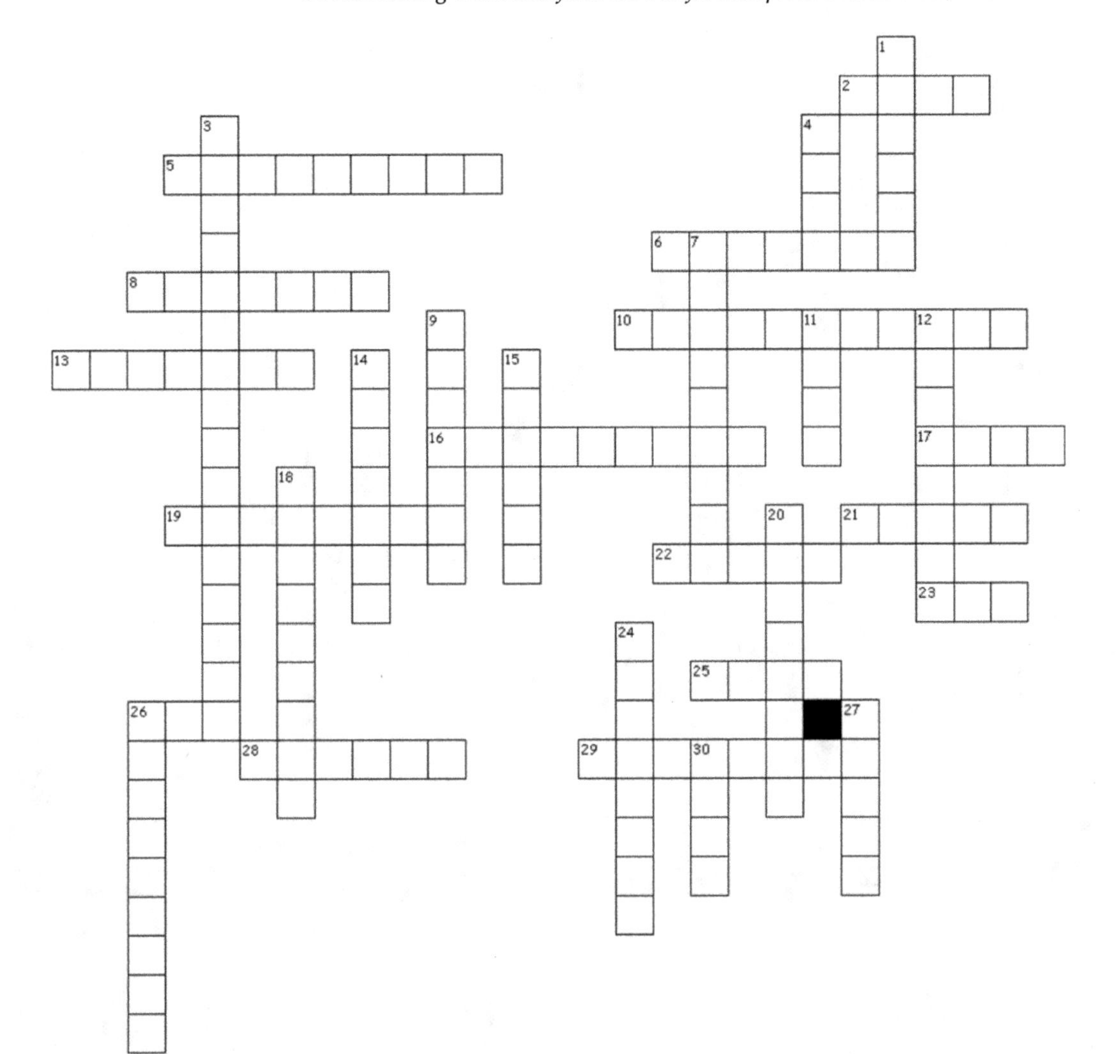

May 2004

47.

The Vocabulary of Cardiology

Crossword Puzzle

Back by popular demand from the puzzle-lovers out there is another crossword puzzle. This one is on the subject of cardiology. Try to fill in the words in the corresponding spaces on the puzzle. All the words are common ones you will hear in cardiology. If you would like to learn more about what these words mean, here's another excellent resource for you:

> **Interpreter's Resource**
>
> Here's a great resource if you come across words whose meaning you do not know. This medical dictionary online is free and easy to use. Check it out!
> http://www.medterms.com

When you are done, try to find either a direct linguistic equivalent or a way to clearly and succinctly explain the term in your non-English language. Have fun!

Across

1. A procedure in which new routes are created around blocked or narrowed coronary arteries, so that increased oxygen and nutrients can get to the heart muscle
4. A thin, flexible tube placed into a blood vessel or body opening to create a pathway for fluids to flow in or out
5. Unpleasant sensations of irregular and/or forceful beating of the heart
9. Swelling
12. Blood that has converted from a liquid to a solid state
13. Abnormal flow of blood through the heart that can be heard on a stethoscope. This abnormality may be of no significance, or it may be very serious.
14. A tube or tiny metal cage designed to be inserted into a vessel or passageway to keep it open
18. The formation of a blood clot in a blood vessel
19. An ultrasound of the heart
21. An irregular heartbeat
22. The blocking of a blood vessel by a foreign substance or blot clot

Down

2. A localized widening of an blood vessel or of the heart. The wall of the vessel is typically weakened and may burst.
3. A procedure used to treat narrowing of the coronary arteries in which a small catheter with a balloon on the end is inserted into the artery of the groin or arm and advanced to narrowing in the coronary artery. The balloon is inflated to enlarge the narrowing, allowing more blood and oxygen to be delivered to the heart muscle.
6. A device imbedded in the heart that generates an electronic pulse to keep the heart beating normally
7. A medication that prevents blood clots
8. The type of cell in the blood that makes it clot
9. A test that measures the electrical activity in the heart
10. The sudden death of brain cells due to lack of oxygen, due to blockage of blood flow or the rupture of an artery in the brain. Also called a cerebrovascular accident or CVA.
11. Forces from the outside world that impact an individual's ability to function. Although a normal part of life that helps us learn and grow, prolonged, uninterrupted, unexpected and unmanageable forms of this can cause significant health problems.
15. Present at birth

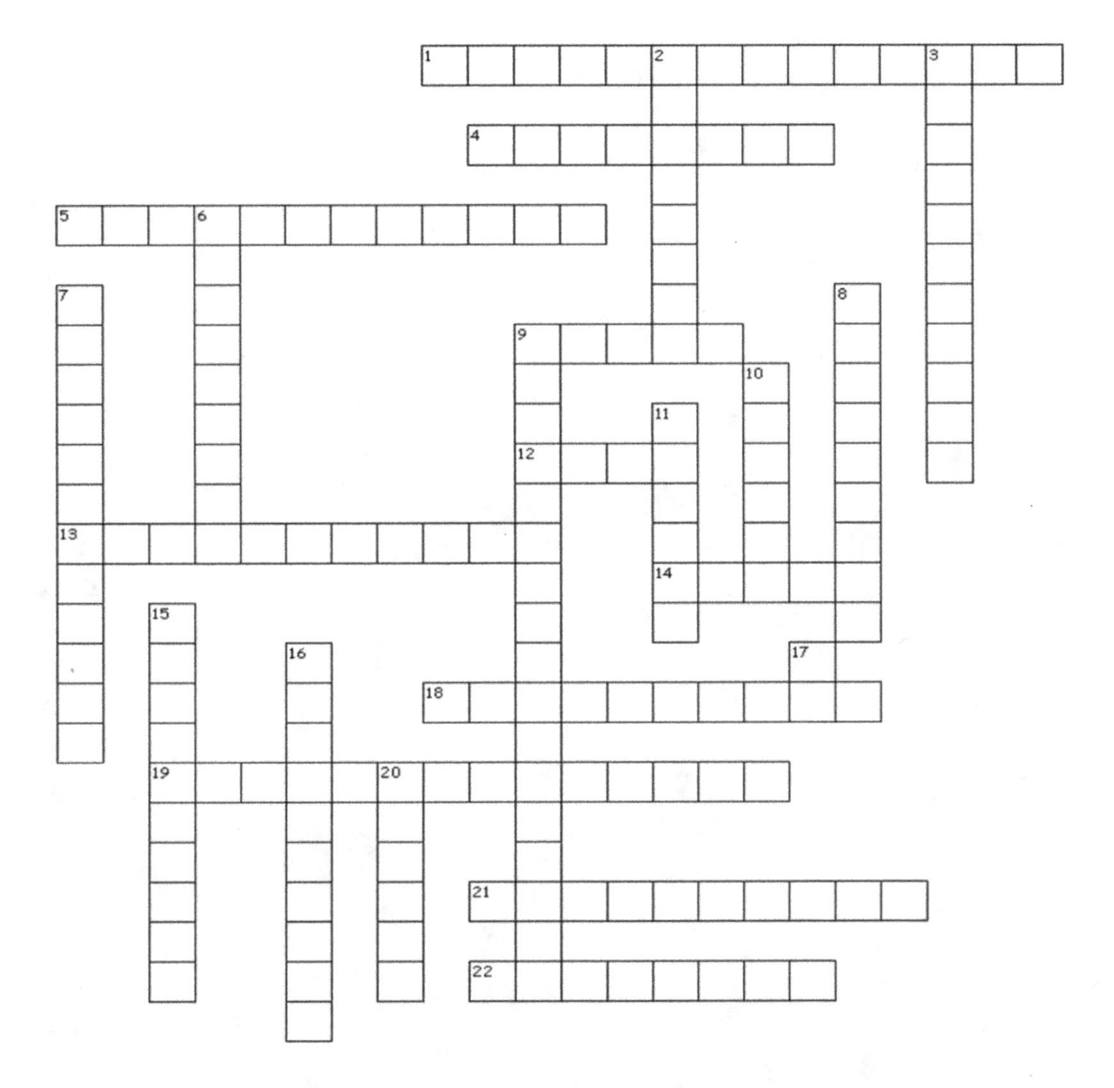

16. The oxygen-carrying pigment and primary protein in red blood cells
17. The acronym used to denote a heart attack
20. Pain in the chest

September 2004

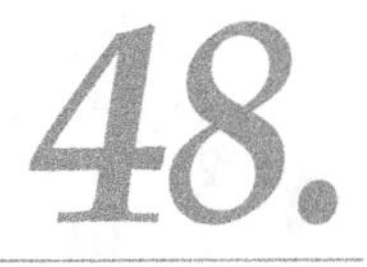

The Muscoloskeletal System

Crossword Puzzle

Here's a chance to "bone up" on some anatomy! Check out this website, especially the parts on the skeleton, the muscles and the nervous system:

http://www.bbc.co.uk/science/humanbody/body/

Across

5. The part of the brain that interprets visual images is the ___________ lobe.
11. The largest part of the brain, located at the top of the head, that is made up of four lobes
12. Lower leg bone, one of two
13. The part of the brain that monitors thirst, hunger, and body temperature, as well as regulating the release of hormones from the pituitary gland
18. Tissue that cushions bones where they rub against other bones
19. The kind of muscles that allow us to move
20. Lower leg bone, one of two
22. When muscles aren't used, they ________________.
23. Structure that allows the body to bend
25. Nugget-like bones in the wrist
26. Tissue that connects bones to bones
27. Lower arm bone, one of two
28. Tailbone
29. The part of the brain that directs sensory signals to the appropriate area in the brain
31. The brain and spinal cord form the __________ nervous system.
32. The part of the brain that regulates unconscious life support functions such as breathing, heartbeat, digestion, blood pressure and sleep
37. Lower arm bone, one of two
38. Tissue that connects bones to muscles (plural)

Down

1. Collar bone
2. The part of the brain that handles speech, thought and emotion is the _________ lobe.
3. The part of the brain that controls muscle movement, balance and posture
4. Flat, triangular bone at the back of the pelvis
6. All the nerves outside the brain and spinal cord form the ___________ nervous system
7. The kind of muscle found only in the heart
8. The part of the brain that interprets auditory impulses and manages memory is the _______ lobe.
9. Heel bone
10. Shoulder blade

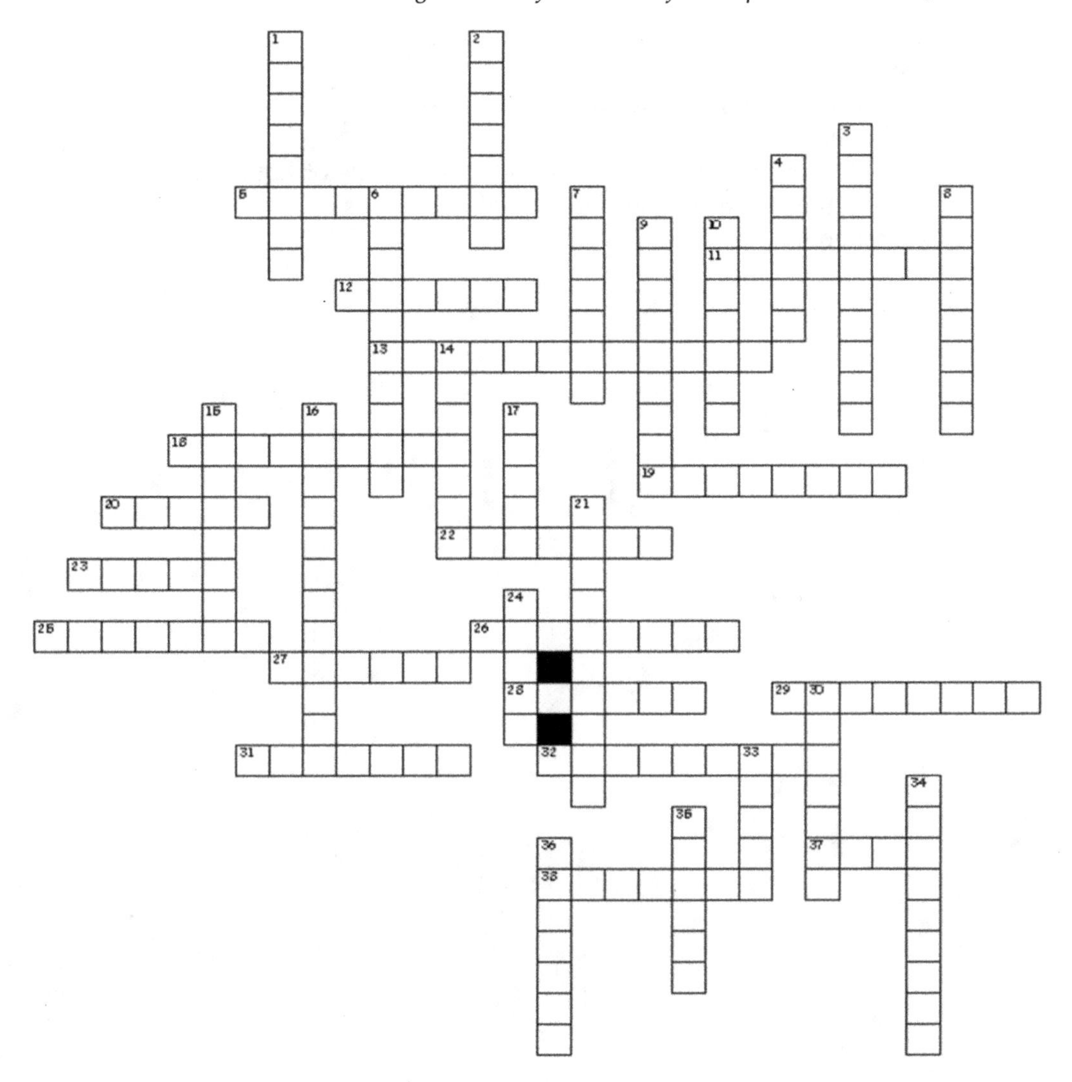

14. Kneecap
15. The part of the brain that handles sensation such as touch, temperature and pain, is the ________ lobe.
16. The part of the brain made up of the thalamus and the hypothalamus
17. Upper leg bone
21. A long, thick bundle of nerves connecting the brain with the rest of the nervous system
24. Round pads of tough cartilage filled with a jelly-like substance that

Continued, next page...

act as shock absorbers and allow the spine to bend

30. Upper arm bone
33. The bone immediately above the heel bone
34. Finger bones
35. The kind of muscles that are found in the walls of hollow organs such as the intestines, the bladder, and the uterus
36. Breast bone

February 2008

49.

Home Health & Safety

Crossword Puzzle

Outdoor activities can lead to new vocabulary needs for interpreters, especially for children during summer vacation. This crossword uses vocabulary related to summer home health and safety. Test your knowledge in English, then find an equivalent term or phrase in your other target language(s).

Across

1. A life-threatening illness in which body temperature rises rapidly; symptoms include dry skin, rapid, strong pulse and dizziness
5. Breathing rapidly
6. A seat with wheels used to take small children for a walk
7. Convulsions
10. A cream or spray that protects the skin from being burned by the sun's ultraviolet rays
13. A protective head covering
14. Fun to watch on the Fourth of July; dangerous to play with
17. What happens to fair skin that is out in the sun too long
18. The state of the joint in a child with "nursemaid's elbow"
23. A child's toy; squishy colored material that can be modeled into different shapes and forms
26. Opposite of awake and aware
27. A dental orthotic used to straighten crooked teeth over a period of months or years
28. A special seat for children, with long legs and a tray in front
29. To be unable to breath due to something being stuck in the throat
30. The name of a graphic icon that is used to designate a poison; recognizable to children
32. An apparatus used in a car that lifts a child higher so the seatbelt fits correctly
35. A child between the ages of two and four
37. The color of bruised skin
38. Designed so that children cannot use it to hurt themselves
39. To lose consciousness
40. An outdoor area with special equipment designated for children to play
41. Thread-like material used to clean between teeth

Down

2. An item of play equipment that children climb up and zoom down
3. A commercially available solution that is used to induce vomiting in someone who has swallowed something poisonous
4. A child-sized portable toilet
6. An abrasion; a superficial injury in which the skin is broken
8. A minor injury resulting from blunt force trauma; looks awful but heals in a few days
9. Skin irritation from excessive sweating

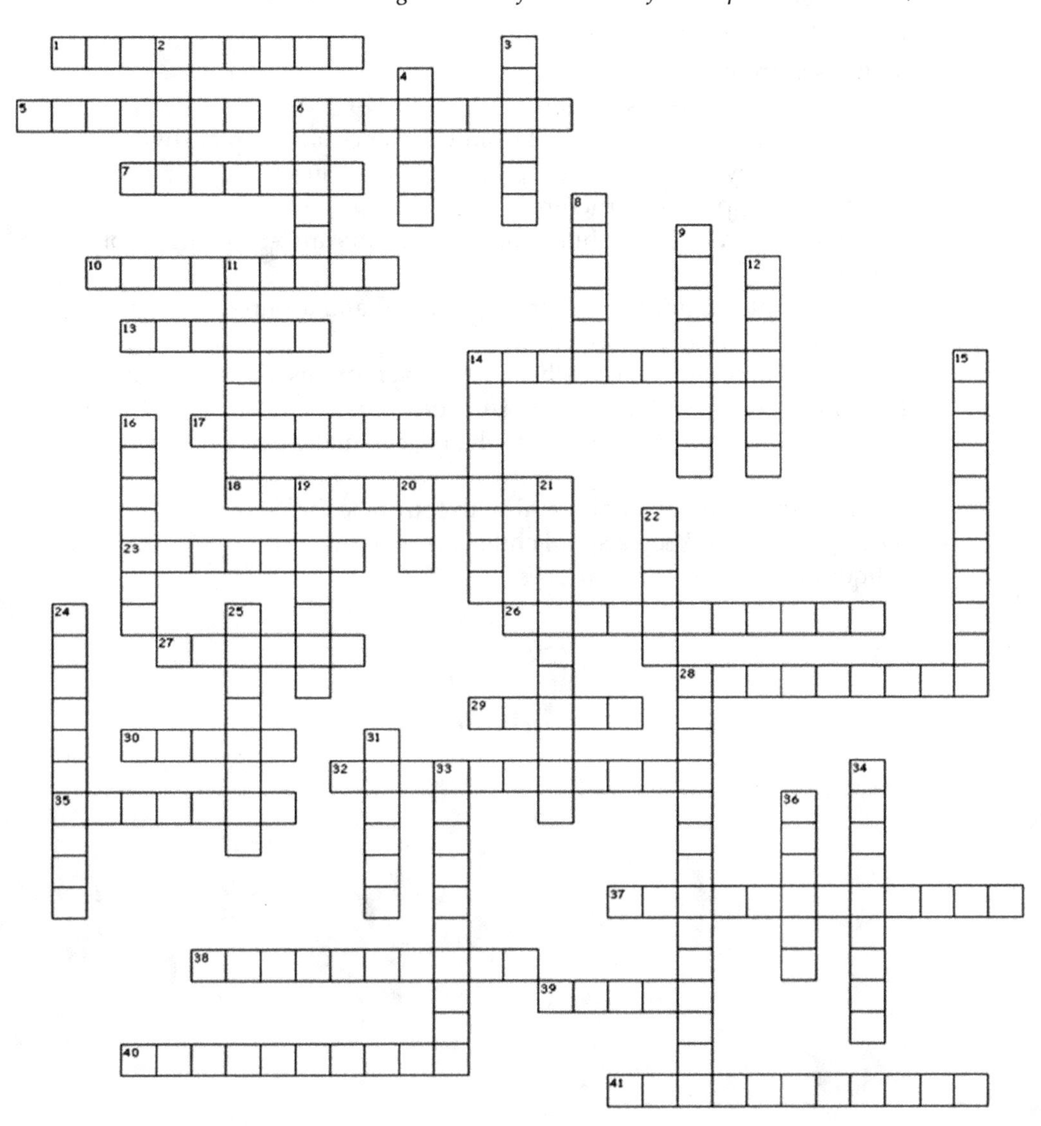

11. A fracture in which part of a bone is protruding from the skin
12. A bubble of clear liquid under the skin, caused by burning or irritation
14. A break in a bone
15. An instrument used to measure a person's temperature
16. A portable enclosure where a child can play safely

Continued, next page...

19. A child's toy made of a flat board with wheels and a pole with handles in front
20. Cardiopulmonary resuscitation
21. A structure at the edge of a pool from which people jump or dive
22. An item of play equipment comprising a seat connected by ropes or chains to a supporting structure
24. A person who cares for a child when the parents are temporarily not available
25. An item of play equipment that goes around and around, on which several children can ride at a time
28. An illness that can precede heatstroke; symptoms include heavy sweating, rapid breathing and a fast, weak pulse
31. Any substance that, if ingested or inhaled, can make people ill or kill them
33. A child's toy made of a flat board with four wheels
34. Sitting in this will keep a small child safe in a car
36. A liquid used to sanitize surfaces

July 2009

50.

The Vocabulary of Nutrition

Crossword Puzzle

These days, it seems like everyone is on a diet! For interpreters, this may mean more nutritional consults. Two great resources for this puzzle and for questions on nutrition in general are http://www.nutrition.gov and the Food and Nutrition Information Center at http://fnic.nal.usda.gov. This latter site even has information on ethnic-specific foods and nutrition that could be helpful to both you and the nutritionists for whom you interpret. Test your knowledge in English, then find an equivalent term or phrase in your other target language(s).

Across

4. A steroid alcohol that supports metabolism; when a constituent of LDL, it may cause arteriosclerosis
5. Bananas have a high level of this mineral.
7. Grown without exposure to chemical fertilizers, growth stimulants, antibiotics or pesticides
8. Found in meat, fish, poultry, dry beans and nuts, the body uses this to build and repair tissue.
10. The amount of heat necessary to raise the temperature of one gram of water from 0° C to 100° C; the amount of food having this energy-producing value
14. A serious eating disorder characterized by obsessive eating followed by purging
15. A dietary ______________; a product that contains vitamins, minerals, herbs or amino acids, that is not considered a food
17. With vitamins or minerals added
19. An agent added to a food to improve color, flavor, texture, or keeping qualities
21. The amount of a particular food eaten at one sitting
24. A mineral found in dairy products and some vegetables; the body uses this to build bones and teeth
26. Animal tissue made up of cells distended with greasy or oily matter
27. Adequate levels of this mineral prevent anemia.
28. A cereal grain that still contains the bran and the germ; generally considered to be healthier
29. The fundamental source of energy for the body

Down

1. Salt
2. A poisonous substance
3. Chemicals added to food so that they don't spoil
6. The chemical changes in living cells by which energy is provided for vital processes
9. Freed from impurities
11. Tasteless
12. The sticky protein substance of wheat flour; some people are allergic to this
13. A substance that provides nutrition

Continued, page 250...

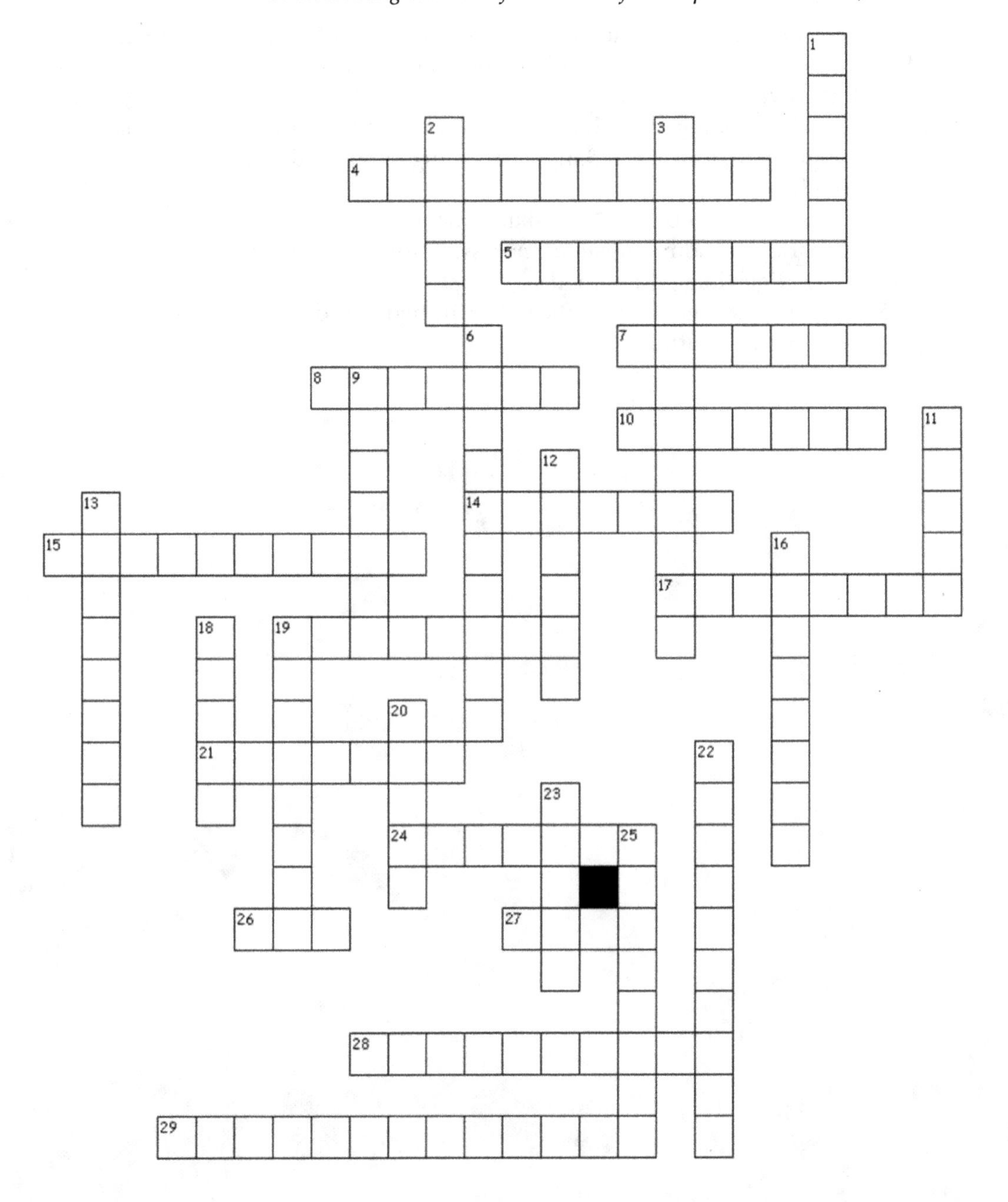
1
2
3
4
5
6
7
8
9
10
11
12
13
14
15
16
17
18
19
20
21
22
23
24
25
26
27
28
29

16. Any of the organic substances naturally occurring in the human body and used in the control of metabolic processes
18. Excessively overweight
19. A serious eating disorder characterized by a pathological fear of weight gain, leading to dangerous eating habits and often excessive weight loss
20. A small amount of food; less than a meal
22. A shortage of some substance necessary for good health
23. The indigestible part of food
25. Any of the inorganic substances that the body needs in trace amounts for optimal health

January 2010

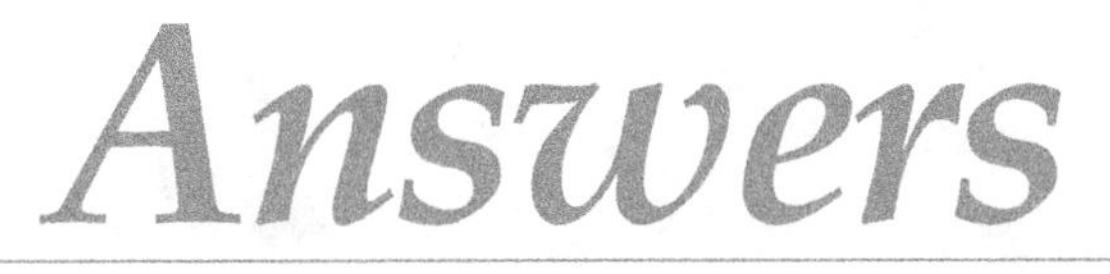

to Exercises & Crossword Puzzles

Chapter 39 – The Vocabulary of Obstetrics

Terms:

6	abortion	22	dilated
11	miscarriage	17	umbilical cord
4	Rh factor	7	preeclampsia
8	Down syndrome	9	episiotomy
12	bag of waters	19	let-down reflex
13	epidural	5	meconium
14	cesarean section	15	amniocentesis
1	fetal distress	16	inverted nipples
2	fetal monitor	10	Corionic Villus Sampling (CVS)
18	breech presentation	20	crowning
21	natural childbirth	23	afterbirth
3	alpha Fetoprotein		

Exercise

Mrs. Green was pleased when she found out she was pregnant again. She had already had two **miscarriages** (one at six weeks and one at three months), and she was a bit afraid that she might not be able to carry to term. She was also a bit surprised that her obstetrician wanted her to have a series of tests, just because she was 38 years old. The first was just a blood test to check for **alpha fetoproteins,** which turned out normal. But when an ultrasound showed mucal thickening, the doctor suggested that she have a **Corionic Villus sampling** to rule out **Down syndrome.** This test showed some abnormalities, but the doctor explained that it might just be the placenta that was affected. So Mrs. Green went back at 14 weeks for an **amniocentesis**. Thank goodness that test came back normal! She also learned that her **Rh factor** was the same as the baby's, which was a relief. Blood tests ruled out gestational diabetes and blood pressure checks ruled out **preeclampsia**.

It was early in the morning, four days before her due date, when Mrs. Green felt her **bag of waters** break. She and her family all went to the hospital. The doctor checked her cervix and found that she was only three centimeters dilated, so she had a while to wait. Over the following hours labor progressed slowly. Mrs. Green had prepared for **natural childbirth** and wanted no drugs or anesthesia, but as the hours wore on, she became very tired. Her obstetrician hooked her up to a **fetal monitor** to see how she and the baby were doing.

After 12 hours of labor, Mrs. Green had dilated to ten centimeters and was finally ready to deliver. The obstetrician did an **episiotomy** so that Mrs. Green would not tear during delivery. Then, as the baby entered the birth canal and started to **crown,** the

fetal monitor suddenly showed the baby entering into **fetal distress**. A resident who was there suggested giving Mrs. Green an **epidural** and doing an emergency **cesarean section** to remove the baby surgically. The obstetrician however, carefully supporting the baby's head, inserted a finger into the birth canal and found that the **umbilical cord** was wrapped around the baby's neck. She slipped it over the baby's head, and the baby was quickly born.

A few minutes later, the **afterbirth** was delivered, and a nurse placed Mrs. Green's new baby girl on her breast. Even though her milk wouldn't **let down** for a while, the baby latched right on and started sucking. The family came in to visit and see their new daughter and sister for the first time.

Chapter 40 – The Vocabulary of Housing Services

Terms:

5	application fee	3	security deposit
13	transitional housing	16	annual review
11	reinstate	17	lease
18	credit check	12	subsidized
24	evaluation	1	evict
19	eligible	7	inspection
10	low-income	15	voucher
14	vacancy	4	food stamps
9	Section 8 housing	20	grievance hearing
21	30-day notice	23	tax-credit-apartment
2	case manager	6	Housing Authority
22	referral	8	pay-or-vacate notice

Exercise

Fatana couldn't find a place to live. It seemed that everywhere she looked, the rents were too expensive. Even with her **food stamps** from the WIC program to help pay for food, she couldn't seem to find enough money to pay for an apartment. And the process of finding an apartment for herself and her family was so complicated! Finally, a social worker gave her a **referral** to the **Housing Authority.**

The Housing Authority helps **low-income** families find a place to live by helping them apply to the government for **Section 8 housing**, for **a tax credit apartment**, or for other **subsidized** housing programs. They often help people who are moving back into general society from **transitional housing**.

After an assessment of Fatana's situation, the Housing Authority determined that she was **eligible** to receive assistance. With help from her **case manager**, Fatana learned about how the housing market works. First she had to wait for a **vacancy** in Section 8 Housing. When an apartment was finally available, the landlord then asked Fatana to fill out an application and to pay an **application fee**. Then he did a **credit check** to see how well Fatana had paid her bills in the past. Once he had approved her application and had reviewed her **voucher**, Fatana had to pay a **security deposit** on the apartment; she was told that if she took good care of the apartment, she'd get this back later. She and the landlord did an **inspection** of the property together, so they would both agree on the condition of the property before she moved in. The landlord asked her to sign a rental agreement (called a **lease**) and explained that she would need to pay her rent on time. If she repeatedly failed to pay her rent, he would send her a **pay or vacate notice**. If she still did not pay, he would send her a **30-day notice**, informing her that he was starting the legal proceedings to have her **evicted**.

After a year, Fatana had an **annual review** and was shocked when she found that the Housing Authority intended to terminate her benefits. She immediately requested a **grievance hearing** to protest her loss of benefits. The Housing Authority did an **evaluation** of her case, and, realizing that they had made a mistake, they **reinstated** her in the program.

Chapter 41 – The Vocabulary of Domestic Abuse

Terms:

2	advocate	8	to file for dissolution
5	Child Protective Services (CPS)	23	confidential shelter
14	safety plan	3	communal setting
18	crisis line	7	cycle of abuse
6	crazy-making	22	survivor
9	domestic violence	13	red flags
10	goals and objectives	19	walking on eggshells
11	intimate partner	1	abuser
12	protection order	20	put-downs
21	victim	15	shelter
4	confidential	17	transitional housing program
16	TANF (Temporary Aid for Needy Families)		

Exercise

Alba was afraid for her life and for the lives of her children. Alba's husband, Raúl, was a violent man. He had hit both her and her children in the past, and this time he had beaten her up so badly that she'd had to go to the hospital. When she was released, she was afraid to go home. She was so tired of **walking on eggshells**, always afraid that something she said might trigger Raúl's violent temper. Even worse, she was afraid that he might start to hit the children, and that the State Office of **Child Protective Services** might take the children away. She was fed up with being a **victim**, accepting anything that Raúl did to her.

So instead of going home, Alba picked up the telephone and called a **crisis line**. The person who answered the phone was trained to help people who were having personal emergencies. This person told Alba about Domestic Abuse Women's Network (DAWN). DAWN is a **shelter** for women and children who are victims of **domestic abuse**. That means that their **intimate partners** abuse them physically and/or psychologically. The people who work at DAWN help women break the **cycle of abuse** by assisting them in becoming independent of the abuser, in becoming **survivors** instead of victims.

When Alba got to the DAWN shelter, she felt safe for the first time in years. This was a **confidential shelter**; nobody could even get the address unless they actually worked there or needed help there. Alba met with an **advocate**, who helped Alba develop **goals and objectives** about what she wanted to happen. This person also helped her develop a **safety plan** for herself and her children so that she would always know how to keep them and herself safe. Her advocate helped Alba file for a **protection order,** (also called a "restraining order" or a "no-contact order"), so that Raúl could not come near her or her children. She also helped Alba apply to the State Medicaid office for **TANF** so that she'd have some income, and to a **transitional housing program** so that she could find her own place to live.

At DAWN, Alba lived in a **communal setting**, together with other women who's been abused and their children. She felt safe there, especially because everything she told her advocate was kept **confidential,** even from the other women at the shelter. She could decide what and when she wanted other people to know about her situation. She did share some things in her women's group, where she learned about the **red flags** that indicate that a man may be an **abuser**. She learned that abuse is more than just physical violence. It includes all the constant **put-downs** she got from Raúl and the **crazy-making** things her husband did on purpose just to make her feel bad. She began to think about whether she should end her marriage by **filing for dissolution**.

Chapter 42 – The Vocabulary of Dentistry

Terms:

18	dental floss	21	prophylaxis
20	calculus	2	root canal
27	extract	16	palate
30	wisdom tooth	10	impacted
5	decay	3	cavity
19	plaque	26	braces
1	bite	12	orthodontist
17	periodontal disease	28	retainer
11	milk teeth	24	dentures
23	pulp	6	sealants
22	crowding	8	fluoride
14	overbite	25	recession
4	gums	13	abscess
9	gingivitis	7	enamel
29	bridge	15	crown

Exercise:

Good morning, Mrs. Hong. I'm Dr. Nguyen. Before we get going on your children's cleaning, I'd like to let you know what we'll be doing today.

Mainly, we'll be doing **prophylaxis** on the children today, to make sure their teeth are nice and clean and to get rid of any **plaque** and **calculus**. Then I'll take a look in their mouths, just to check for possible **cavities.** We'll apply a **fluoride** treatment, to protect the **enamel** on the teeth, and on the two older children, we'll also be putting **sealant** on their molars to protect against **decay**.

Now, about your youngest daughter, May; I see that her **milk teeth** are beginning to fall out and that she's getting her adult teeth. There seems to be a fair bit of **crowding**, so I think you should be prepared that she will probably need **braces** when she's a bit older to straighten the teeth out and to correct her **bite**. I'll refer you to an **orthodontist** when the time comes. We'll probably want to **extract** her **wisdom teeth** too, when they start to come in, since there probably won't be enough room for them. Unless they are **impacted**, that's a fairly simple procedure.

Now let's talk about your dental needs for a moment. First of all, the X-rays showed that there is a very deep **cavity** in this tooth here and that the **pulp** has become badly infected. It's beginning to form an **abscess**. I'll bet that hurts a lot. We're going to need to do a **root canal**, but first I'd like to treat the infection with an antibiotic. After we clean out the **cavity**, control the infection and do the **root canal**, I'll put a **crown** on the tooth.

Secondly, I can see that you're getting some **recession** of the **gums** - see here where the root of the tooth is beginning to show? You can stop this process by a using **dental floss** every day. That will also help you lower your risk here of **periodontal disease**.

Finally, I see you're missing a tooth back here. As a result, the neighboring teeth are shifting out of their correct placement. Have you thought about getting a **bridge**? That would help the teeth stay in the right place.

Chapter 43 – The Vocabulary of the Business Office

Terms:

10	occupation	19	pre-existing condition
17	spouse	9	certificate of coverage
27	insurance	20	COBRA
1	policy	18	Federal Poverty Level
30	work-related injury	29	fee-for-service
11	medical record	2	low income
22	next-of-kin	28	Medicaid
6	benefits	21	Medicare
12	co-pay	5	managed care
8	deductible	15	partner
13	eligible	3	WIC (Women, Infants and Children)
25	coinsurance	14	power of attorney
23	retroactive	4	primary care provider
24	advanced directive	26	prior authorization review
16	appeal	7	SSI (Supplemental Security Income)

Chapter 44 – Idioms, Acronyms & Abbreviations

Idioms

1.	above all	most importantly
2.	as fit as a fiddle	very healthy
3.	as good as gold	very good, well-behaved
4.	as hungry as a bear	very hungry
5.	as regular as clockwork	always at the same time
6.	as sharp as a tack	very aware, intelligent
7.	as sick as a dog	very sick

8. baloney	nonsense; an untrue statement or opinion
9. to beat around the bush	to waste time by not giving a direct answer
10. bed of roses	comfortable; an easy situation
11. to break the ice	to begin a conversation, for instance, with a stranger
12. a breeze	very easy thing to do
13. bushed	very tired, exhausted
14. come rain or shine	regardless of the circumstances
15. to cost an arm and a leg	to be very expensive
16. down the drain	wasted, lost
17. to eat like a horse	to eat a lot
18. fair and square	honestly, without cheating
19. to feel blue	to feel sad; to be depressed
20. for the time being	temporarily
21. forty winks	a short sleep, a nap
22. get a kick out of something	to enjoy something a lot
23. to go bananas	to get very excited; go crazy
24. to give the green light	to approve
25. in a nutshell	in a few words; in summary
26. in a pickle	in trouble
27. in seventh heaven	extremely happy
28. in the nick of time	just before it is too late
29. in the same boat	in the same situation
30. ins and outs	(the) details
31. to keep the ball rolling	to make something continue to happen
32. the last straw	the last thing in a series of bad things that finally makes someone become angry
33. a long face	a sad appearance
34. to make a mountain out of a molehill	to exaggerate a small problem
35. to nip something in the bud	to stop something when it's just beginning
36. no dice	no; not approved; not permitted
37. on pins and needles	very nervous or excited when expecting something
38. on the ball	alert and aware
39. on the fence	undecided; unwilling or unable to make a decision

40. on the house	free; without cost, as a gift
41. once in a blue moon	very seldom; almost never
42. out of the blue	by surprise; unexpectedly
43. out of the woods	free from difficulty or danger, after a difficult period or situation
44. pain in the neck	something or someone that is annoying
45. to pan out	to succeed
46. a piece of cake	very easy to do
47. to pull someone's leg	to fool someone in a joking manner
48. to put the cards on the table	to explain something or some situation completely and honestly
49. to put two and two together	to come to a conclusion; to figure something out
50. red tape	complicated procedures; bothersome rules and regulations; forms and papers to fill out
51. to run in the family	to be characteristic of many family members
52. second nature	easy and natural to do
53. to see eye to eye	to understand and agree (about something) with another person
54. sink or swim	fail or succeed
55. sixth sense	a special feeling or intuition; a feeling that something may happen
56. spick-and-span	very clean
57. to take pains	to be sure to do something even if it is difficult
58. the tip of the iceberg	a small thing that indicates a larger problem
59. under the weather	sick; not feeling well
60. a white lie	a lie (false statement) that does not cause serious concern or harm

Acronyms

61. AIDS	Acquired Immune Deficiency Syndrome
62. AMA	against Medical Advice
63. BM	bowel Movement
64. BMI	body Mass Index
65. ABG	coronary artery bypassgGraft
66. CT (as in CT Scan)	computed tomography
67. CBC	complete blood count

68. COPD — chronic obstructive pulmonary disease
69. ECG — electrocardiogram
70. EEG — electroencephalogram
71. EMG — electromyogram
72. GERD — gastroesophageal reflux disease
73. GVHD — Graft-vs.-Host Disease
74. HIV — human immunodeficiency virus
75. HPV — human papiloma virus
76. IUD — intrauterine device
77. IVP — intravenous pyelography (or pyelogram)
78. MI — myocardial Infarction
79. MRI — magnetic resonance imaging
80. NICU — Neonatal Intensive Care Unit
81. NPO — nothing by mouth
82. NSAID — nonsteroidal anti-inflammatory drug
83. PCP — primary care provider
84. R_X — prescription
85. T_X — treatment
86. URI — upper respiratory infection
87. UTI — urinary tract infection

Language Access Acronyms

88. OCR — Office for Civil Rights
89. ATA — American Translators Association
90. CHIA — California Healthcare Interpreting Association
91. DHHS — Department of Health and Human Services
92. DOJ — Department of Justice
93. IMIA — International Medical Interpreter Association
94. IS — interpreter services
95. LAC — language access coordinator
96. LEP — limited English proficient
97. LLD — language of limited diffusion
98. NCIHC — National Council on Interpreting in Health Care
99. OPI — over the phone interpreting

Chapter 45 – Slang Vocabulary & Exercises

Terms:

6	ahead of the game	21	back to square one
20	to backfire	24	bang for the buck
5	bells and whistles	16	to bite the bullet
22	to buy time	11	to call the shots
1	catch-22	19	Check it out
18	close call	23	to cut down on
2	give us a ring	17	to go through the proper channels
9	goofed	3	hop up here
7	I take it	13	lickety-split
10	to pull something off	4	to rule out
14	to run in the family	12	to slip on
8	tah-dah!	15	X marks the spot.

Exercise

Mr. Sanchez, I know you don't want people to think you're disabled, but you're just going to have to **bite the bullet** and use a cane.

We should have the results next week. Why don't you **give me a ring** and I'll go over them with you?

We thought that telling your Mom that she needs to do her exercises so that you all don't have to come take care of her every day would get her motivated, but the plan **backfired**; now she won't even try to do the exercises!

Let me give you a prescription for the 800 mg. pills instead of the 200 mg. They have more **bang for the buck**.

You are so lucky - you're getting the newest birthing suite in the hospital. It's got all the **bells** and whistles.

This treatment isn't going to cure the cancer, but it will **buy** us **some time**.

We were going to wait to start the next round of chemotherapy, but you've responded so well so far that we're planning on starting next week. That way we'll be **ahead of the game.**

I need to ask what your parents died of, because some health problems **run in the family.**

You're stuck in a real **catch-22.** If you go back to work, you'll lose your Medicaid, but if you don't go back to work, you won't be able to afford the co-pay for your services here. I'm not sure what to advise you!

I can only give you my opinion, Mrs. Nguyen; you and your family are the ones who are **calling the shots**.

Here on the ultrasound, you can see your baby, Mrs. Gorchenko. Hey, **check it out,** here's her little foot!

I need you to tell me exactly where your knee hurts, so tell me if it hurts as I press here. . . or here. . . or here. . or – ah hah! **X marks the spot**!

It's a good thing you brought him in when you did. He was bleeding heavily internally. It was **a close call**. Any later and I don't think we could have saved him.

Regarding your diet, you absolutely must **cut down** on the amount of salt you're eating. It's not good for your blood pressure.

I don't know if the hospital will give you a discount or not. We'll have to **go through the proper channels** and see what they say.

Oops, I **goofed**.

Let's get that cast right off, and we'll have you out of here **lickety-split**.

All the tests came back negative. As far as figuring out what you have, we're **back to square one.**

We usually don't use the laparoscope to do the surgery when the patient is in the middle of a gall bladder attack, but we gave it a try and we **pulled it off**.

This test will help us **rule out** the possibility that the lump is cancer.

So, **I take it** you don't feel the medication helped any.

Why don't you just **slip on** this gown and **hop up here** on the exam table so that I can take a look at that shoulder?

So, we take the bandages off and – **tah dah**! You can see!

Chapter 46 – Signs & Symptoms

Across
2. Sore
5. Dizziness
6. Tremble
8. Seizure
10. Constipated
13. Fatigue
16. Twitching
17. Glum
19. Wheezing
21. Stiff
22. Fever
23. Gas
25. Weak
26. Pus
28. Cramps
29. Diarrhea

Down
1. Hoarse
3. Ringing in the ears
4. With no feeling
7. Runny nose
9. Vertigo
11. Itch
12. Tingling
14. Flaking
15. Shiver
18. Heartburn
20. Headache
24. Vomiting
26. Premature
27. Faint
30. Rash

Chapter 47 – The Vocabulary of Cardiology

Across
1. Coronary bypass
4. Catheter
5. Palpitations
9. Edema
12. Clot
13. Heart murmur
14. Stent
18. Thrombosis
19. Echocardiogram
21. Arrhythmia
22. Embolism

Down
2. Aneurysm
3. Angioplasty
6. Pacemaker
7. Blood thinner
8. Platelet
9. Electrocardiogram
10. Stroke
11. Stress
15. Congenital
16. Hemoglobin
17. MI
20. Angina

Chapter 48 – The Musculoskeletal System

Across

5. Occipital
11. Cerebrum
12. Fibula
13. Hypothalamus
18. Cartilage
19. Skeletal
20. Tibia
22. Atrophy
23. Joint
25. Carpals
26. Ligament
27. Radius
28. Tailbone
29. Thalamus
31. Central
32. Brain stem
37. Ulna
38. Tendons

Down

1. Clavical
2. Frontal
3. Cerebellum
4. Sacrum
6. Peripheral
7. Cardiac
8. Temporal
9. Calcaneus
10. Scapula
14. Patella
15. Parietal
16. Diencephalon
17. Femur
21. Spinal cord
24. Discs
30. Humerus
33. Talus
34. Phalanges
35. Smooth
36. Sternum

Chapter 49 – Home Health & Safety Terms

Across

1. Sunstroke
5. Panting
6. Stroller
7. Seizure
10. Sunscreen
13. Helmet
14. Fireworks
17. Sunburn
18. Dislocated
23. Play-Doh
26. Unconscious
27. Braces
28. Highchair
29. Choke
30. Mr. Yuk
32. Booster seat
35. Toddler
37. Black and blue
38. Childproof
39. Faint
40. Playground
41. Dental floss

Down

2. Slide
3. Ipecac
4. Potty
6. Scrape
8. Bruise
9. Heat rash
11. Compound
12. Blister
14. Fracture
15. Thermometer
16. Playpen
19. Scooter
20. CPR
21. Diving board
22. Swing
24. Babysitter
25. Carousel
28. Heat exhaustion
31. Poison
33. Skateboard
34. Child seat
36. Bleach

Chapter 50 – The Vocabulary of Nutrition

Across
4. Cholesterol
5. Potassium
7. Organic
8. Protein
10. Calorie
14. Bulimia
15. Supplement
17. Enriched
19. Additive
21. Serving
24. Calcium
26. Fat
27. Iron
28. Whole Grain
29. Carbohydrates

Down
1. Sodium
2. Toxin
3. Preservatives
6. Metabolism
9. Refined
11. Bland
12. Gluten
13. Nutrient
16. Vitamins
18. Obese
19. Anorexia (technically, anorexia nervosa)
20. Snack
22. Deficiency
23. Fibre
25. Minerals

CPSIA information can be obtained
at www.ICGtesting.com
Printed in the USA
LVHW100800101220
673651LV00024B/229